A STUDY OF
THE ENGLISH APOTHECARY
FROM 1660 TO 1760

(*Medical History*, Supplement No. 3, 1983)

DEDICATION

To the memory of my mother, Amy Kathleen Thomas.

A STUDY OF
THE ENGLISH APOTHECARY
FROM 1660 TO 1760

by

JUANITA G. L. BURNBY

(*Medical History*, Supplement No. 3)

LONDON

WELLCOME INSTITUTE FOR THE HISTORY OF MEDICINE

1983

Published 1983 by the Wellcome Institute for the History of Medicine, 183 Euston Road, London NW1 2BP.

ISBN 0 85484 043 5
ISSN   0025 7273 3

Supplements to *Medical History* may be obtained at the Wellcome Institute, or by post from Science History Publications Ltd, Halfpenny Furze, Chalfont St Giles, Bucks HP8 4NR, England.

Printed by the Wellcome Foundation Limited, Print and Packaging Division (Crewe).

CONTENTS

ACKNOWLEDGMENTS

It is impossible to name more than a few of those who have helped me over the course of many years, but I would like particularly to acknowledge my debt to Miss Margaret Mackenzie who set me on the path of serious historical research, and to Miss Barbara Fenwick who has sat in record offices for many long hours transcribing material for me. Dr Jessie Ridge and Mr F. H. Rawlings have been so generous as to allow me access to their unpublished material, which was extremely useful; whilst the help, encouragement, and stimulating exchange of ideas with Dr Edwin Clarke and Dr Douglas Whittet have proved invaluable. I am very conscious of the debt I owe to the editorial staff of *Medical History*, in particular to Mrs J. Runciman whose patience and ingenuity in dealing with problems seem to be inexhaustible.

To my husband I can but say "Thank you" and that without you none of this work would have been possible.

NOTE

It should be noted that dates of days from the 1st January to the 24th March prior to 1752 are given according to the moden calendrical style, as if the year began on the 1st January.

INTRODUCTION

Numerous papers have been written on individual apothecaries, men of the calibre of Samuel Dale (1659–1739) or W. T. Brande (1788–1866), and apothecaries *per se* have warranted a small section in any book devoted to a general history of medicine, but there is no study in depth of the profession in the important years between the Restoration and the Act of 1815. Still less work has been done on the provincial apothecary of England and Wales. Pharmaceutical history, until recently, has commanded but little attention, and most of that has dealt with London, but, as Trease has written, "To complete the picture we must study not only London records but those from the Continent and our provincial towns. Local pharmaceutical history is as yet a neglected field but one well worth cultivating. We may then obtain answers to such questions as, how numerous were apothecaries in the provinces, and how did their training, practice and financial position compare with London colleagues. . . . Material from a single county may seem trivial but collected and studied for the country as a whole it should add much to our present knowledge."[1]

This study of the English apothecary has three main features – synthesis, social history, and reassessment. The apothecary was a multidisciplinary man; material relating to him may be found in out-of-the-way journals and books of limited circulation, material that must be collected together in order to create a more truly rounded person. His expertise over a wide scientific spectrum was of value and led him into a deep involvement with the new medical and paramedical specializations. As a man of science he played his part. He was intimately concerned in the Scientific Revolution and made considerable contributions to the emerging disciplines of botany and chemistry, as well as to medicine itself. His effect on the development of the general practitioner, the druggist, both wholesale and retail, the chemist, both experimental and manufacturing, and the dispensing pharmacist was enormous but to date none of this has been systematically investigated.

The background, work, and life of those apothecaries who have made a mark in the world, primarily the scientific world, have in some degree been investigated and further facts are not difficult to elucidate, but the story is different for the "ordinary run-of-the-mill chap". His activities and position in the community have been but rarely scrutinized. The Thomas Botts of Coventry or the Lewis Dickensons of Stafford made no mark in the worlds of science or the arts; they were not members of any of the societies then beginning to emerge, but they were the very men who formed the warp and woof of the apothecarial cloth in the busy market towns of England. Knowledge of their lives promotes an understanding and explanation, not only of their training and expertise, but of the community in which they lived. Their friends and relatives, their interests, and their account books all serve to delineate the picture. This type of detailed investigation of apothecaries' lives shows that their social origins were frequently far higher than has been generally allowed, and that their status within their own community was enviable. Monetarily, their position was often sound

---

[1] F. N. L. Poynter (editor), *The evolution of pharmacy in Britain,* London, Pitman Medical Publications, 1965, presidential address by G. E. Trease, p. 11.

1

and an examination of the apprenticeship premiums shows that they belonged to the more favoured sections of the community. Their educational standards and the opportunities they had to obtain this education are important to the realization of the apothecaries' position, some idea of which may be garnered from contemporary letters and memoranda. Self-education was undoubtedly necessary, with the result that many apothecaries retained a keen interest in spheres not directly related to the winning of mere bread and butter; many, in fact, can be regarded as cultured men.

Holmes, in a recent study of the professions in England 1680–1730, a period lying almost squarely within my own, writes that "... far too little is known about their members, either as individuals, or occupational groups or as social entities."[2] The question immediately arises as to whether the apothecary may be regarded as a professional man. Just what constitutes a profession is open to debate. We talk of a professional musician or a professional cricketer when we mean one who earns his livelihood by the playing of music or cricket; on the other hand, we use the term professional engineer to separate one of higher education and recognized qualifications from a turner or fitter, electrician or mechanic. In the present context, a profession can be seen as an occupation that demands that its members must have a good education and be orientated towards a particular career specialization; their expertise must be particularly valued by the community. Further, "a profession" implies a notion of service to the community, a vocation, such as the administration of justice, defence of one's country, or efforts to improve spiritual and physical well-being. Finally, this image is projected by a professional body with powers of registration, supervision, and regulation. Holmes believes that "... such concepts as these were not alien to the seventeenth and early eighteenth century Englishman", but does admit that "... even the major and indisputable professional groups of Augustan England must have had difficulty in experiencing anything resembling a common 'professional' solidarity."[3] In fact Holmes does not go far enough in trying to define the professions, as he places insufficient emphasis on standards and, more importantly, the framing of a code of ethics. He has also a too innocent belief in the powers of enforcement of the regulatory bodies, or their desire to do so. Turning a blind eye was almost a full-time occupation in those years. For these reasons one cannot say, in the modern sense, that the professions were fully fledged by 1760.

The apothecary and his close companion, the surgeon, of the century between 1660 and 1760 do not fulfil all the criteria of professionalism. Their work certainly demanded skill and academic knowledge acquired mainly from apprenticeship but also through books and latterly often by attending courses of lectures. In London, they had to satisfy their companies' courts of assistants that they had a sufficiently high standard of education to commence training, and at the end of their term to pass an examination. To what extent these standards were enforced in the provinces we have no proof, but there is evidence that provincial guilds in some cities at an earlier period were insistent on a standard being maintained. Education and training were by no means uniform throughout the country, or even from master to master, as Crabbe

[2] Geoffrey Holmes, *Augustan England. Professions, state, and society, 1680–1730*, London, Allen & Unwin, 1982, preface, p. x.
[3] Ibid., pp. 3, 7.

so bitterly complained. Qualifications were not easily identifiable, ranging from the frequently ludicrous bishop's licence of the surgeons to the considerably more searching one of the London Society of Apothecaries, to say nothing of hurried trips to the Continent for medical degrees, or those so easily handed out by the universities of Aberdeen and St Andrews.

As to the legalities, it would seem that, despite bitter complaints by all parties, a medical practitioner, were he self-styled physician, surgeon, or apothecary, could practise illegally with a fair degree of impunity in small towns, boroughs, cities, and even the metropolis itself. Whatever royal charter or act of Parliament had been obtained to give a body legal recognition, its enforcement was quite another matter in the absence of any adequate regulatory machinery. Because no registers were kept, it was impossible for a man to be the equivalent of "defrocked" or "struck off". Indeed, all the medical bodies, the College of Physicians not excluded, showed a greater concern with the maintenance of standards for their own wellbeing than for that of the patients, with etiquette rather than ethics.

It was not until some fifty years after our period that it was recognized that the adherence to standards set up for the benefit of the profession and for the patient was inseparable and essential. Nevertheless, the concept of professionalism was growing during the years from 1660 to 1760. There was an increase in self-awareness, of the importance of the apothecary and surgeon to the community, and of their place within it, which led to an increasing degree of group cohesiveness and pride in their occupations. William Boghurst, when writing of his experiences in the Great Plague, gave as his view that those apothecaries who acted as physicians were "... bound by their undertakings to stay and help as in other disease. Every man that undertakes to bee of a profession or takes upon him any office must take all parts of it, the good and the evill, the pleasure and the pain, the profit and the inconvenience altogether, and not pick and chuse; for ministers must preach, Captains must fight, Physitians attend upon the sick, etc."[4] Nearly a century later, young Tom Harris wrote a letter of commiseration to his friend Richard Pulteney, another apothecary apprentice, who had recently been turned over from his Loughborough master to a Mr Wylde in Nottingham. He pitied him for being "... as it were debarred from the Society of the Brothers of your profession", and then added, "I assure you I have conceived a very indifferent idea of your Nottingham gent. and am afraid the sons of physic pay more adoration at the Courts of Venus than those of Aesculapius and I am apt to believe a Rochester or a Cotton would take place before a Mead or Huxam [*sic*]."[5]

The idea of professional responsibility was gaining ground, and if the medical practitioner of 1660 or 1760 cannot be said to have belonged to a profession, it would not be inaccurate to say that he belonged to a proto-profession, whether he were apothecary, surgeon, or physician.

The apothecary was more than just a medical practitioner; he also sold medicaments and chemicals, and dispensed prescriptions. He fulfilled an essential role in his society. Without doubt, both his position and his contribution to the community have been greatly undervalued.

[4] W. Boghurst, *Loimographia, an account of the Great Plague of London in the year 1665*, edited by J. F. Payne, London, Shaw, 1894, p. 59.
[5] Linnean Society, Pulteney letters, letter from Thomas Harris to Richard Pulteney, 15 June 1752.

I

THE PLACE OF THE APOTHECARY IN THE EVOLUTION OF MEDICAL PRACTICE

"WE have to deal here with a sort of men not of Academical, but Mechanick education; who being either actually engaged in the late Rebellion, or bred up in some mean and contemptible trades were never taught the duty they owe to God or their Sovereign, to their Native Country or the Laws therof" – thus wrote Charles Goodall, the energetic defender of the rights of the London College of Physicians, in 1684. Goodall, who became president of the College, had, in 1665, received at Cambridge a licence merely to practise surgery and did not gain incorporation until five years later on the strength of a Leiden MD obtained after a mere thirteen days at that university.[6] In his character assassination of the apothecaries, he was following the example of another fellow of the College, a man of greater stature, Christopher Merrett FRS, who, fourteen years earlier, wrote in his *A short view of the frauds and abuses committed by Apothecaries . . . ,* "But before I descend to particulars I shall first lay down this Proposition. . . . That they may be the Veriest Knaves in England."

These were but two of the many blasts in the pamphlet war between the physicians of the College and the apothecaries of the London Society that raged for the forty years between 1665 and 1705. On the whole, one gains the impression that the opponents were fairly evenly matched, with the weight coming down rather more on the physicians' side. It is a different story from the first phase of the battle immediately before the outbreak of the Civil War, when the position of the Company of Apothecaries was indeed parlous.

The foundation of the College of Physicians dates from 23 September 1518, when Henry VIII granted letters patent under the Great Seal for the incorporation of "the College of Commonalty of the Faculty of Medicine of London". No one was to practise physic within London and for seven miles around unless admitted by the president and College by letters sealed with their common seal, and offenders were to be punished by fines and imprisonment. There was no clause safeguarding the rights of the English universities to be licensing bodies for the practice of physic throughout the kingdom. This was to lead to considerable controversy. Nor was the Act of 1511 repealed. This stated that within London and seven miles around no person was to practise as physician or surgeon unless he were examined and approved by the bishop of London or the dean of St Paul's, who were to be assisted in the case of physicians by four doctors of physic, and in the case of surgeons by experts in surgery. In the rest of the country, aspiring surgeons and physicians were to be examined by the bishop of the diocese or the bishop's vicar-general, who were also to seek assistance from such experts as they thought necessary.

Clark is of the opinion that the ecclesiastical authorities must have regarded their powers as having been revoked in London in respect of physicians, as there was little

---

[6] A. H. T. Robb-Smith, 'Cambridge medicine', in A. G. Debus (editor), *Medicine in seventeenth century England*, Los Angeles, University of California Press, 1974, p. 365.

4

controversy between the bishops and the College, unlike that between the bishops and the surgeons.[7] No Parliament met until 1523, when the College took the opportunity of petitioning for incorporation by statute. The Act (14 & 15 Henry VIII c. 5) was passed without difficulty, a clause being added which greatly extended the College's powers, at least in theory. In the provincial dioceses, it was not always possible to find men capable of examining candidates for the practice of physic as demanded by the Act of 1511, so it was enacted that no one was to practise throughout England until such time as he had been examined at London by the president and three elects and received letters testimonial. The only exceptions were graduates of Oxford and Cambridge who had fulfilled all the requirements for a medical degree without being excused any part. The College's very small numbers and lack of administrative organization outside London made the clause completely ineffective, though it is probable that in it lay the origin of the type of membership known at a later date as "extra-licentiate".

The Act of 1540 increased the powers of the College over the London apothecaries, who at that time were still members of the powerful Grocers' Company, by giving it the right to enter the shop of any apothecary, examine his wares, and, if they were found defective, summon the wardens of that company for their destruction. If we consider that the next Act but one of Henry VIII's reign (32 Hy. VIII c. 42) dealt with the amalgamation of the Barbers' Company and the unincorporated surgeons, they had the remarkable foresight to have included in their Act (32 Hy. VIII c. 40) a clause that any member of the College had the right to practise surgery if he so desired, "Forasmuch as the science of physick doth comprehend, include and contain the knowledge of surgery". They thus safeguarded themselves from possible future accusations of infringing the rights of a City company.

The physicians gained greater coercive powers in the time of Mary, and in the early years of Elizabeth's reign were very active in their efforts to supervise apothecaries' wares. Only days before the sealing of the Bill for the separation of the apothecaries from the grocers, the physicians obtained a new charter from James I which gave them all the powers they wished for controlling non-collegiate practitioners, sellers, and handlers of physic, such as apothecaries, druggists, and distillers. This charter was, however, never confirmed by statute, which the physicians were to find distinctly inhibiting as the Civil War approached.

The desire of the apothecaries to separate from the grocers became apparent in 1588 when they unsuccessfully petitioned the queen to give them a monopoly in the compounding and selling of drugs and medicines; at the same time they accused the physicians of compounding physic. Following the accession of James I, the Company was given a new charter and, in 1606, was explicitly re-incorporated as "The Freemen of the Misteries of Grocers and Apothecaries of the City of London". Despite this title, the apothecaries were still aggrieved, as they had no representation on the governing body of the Company and so could not control their own "mistery".[8] It is possible that their wish to break away had less to do with their concern for the wellbe-

[7] Sir George N. Clark, *A history of the Royal College of Physicians of London*, Oxford, Clarendon Press, 1964, vol. 1, p. 60.

[8] C. Wall, H. C. Cameron, and E. A. Underwood, *A history of the Worshipful Society of the Apothecaries of London*, Oxford University Press, 1963, vol. 1, p. 10.

ing of patients and pharmacy, than with an attempt to escape the dominance of the powerful oligarchic trading elements of the Grocers' Company. The concentration of executive and electoral power in a few hands in the different companies represented the dominance of the merchants over the craft interests. The history of each of the new companies, for example, the felt-makers, the glovers, and the pin-makers, began in the revolt of a craft, or what Unwin calls an industrial section, against the governing body of one of the older companies who were accused of usurping power.[9]

After an unsuccessful Bill in 1610, the apothecaries made another attempt in April 1614, largely at the instigation of Gideon Delaune, apothecary to the queen. This time they petitioned the king, pointing out the dangers that arose from unskilful persons making and selling "... without restraint false and corrupt medicines in and about London...". The petition was well received. The law officers of the Crown, Sir Francis Bacon and Sir Henry Yelverton, were instructed to discuss the matter with the king's physicians, Sir Theodore Turquet de Mayerne and Dr Henry Atkins. On 13 May 1614, it was recommended that the apothecaries should be allowed to separate themselves, because of "... disorders ... many and great ... which wee doe impute partly for the want of skill in the Grocers concearn-inge the Art of the Apothecaries, and partly to the disp[osi]tions incident to marchants and tradesmen rather to favour the Lucrative part of the trade of undersellinge than the true use thereof, by utteringe that, that is perfect and good". The apothecaries, they added, would be more fittingly subordinated to the physicians than merchants and tradesmen. The king accepted this advice.

The first draft of the charter was drawn up, signed by Atkins, Mayerne, and seventy-six apothecaries, and submitted on 23 May 1614 to a comitia of the College of Physicians, where it was approved by a majority. There were twenty clauses, nine of which were concerned with the control of pharmacy. The most notable of the draft recommendations were that there should be no difference in status between freemen who were wholesalers and those engaged in retail pharmacy, and that no apothecary should be allowed to practise unless he had undergone a seven-year apprenticeship and been examined and approved by both the College and the Company, and, further-more, been granted a licence to keep a shop. Pharmacy was to be controlled by the College of Physicians and the new Company within the City and seven miles around, and registers were to be kept of licensed physicians and apothecaries. All apothecaries' shops were to be inspected at least quarterly by the president and censors of the College and the master and wardens of the Company, either separately or together. No by-laws were to be made without the participation in Apothecaries' Hall of the president and censors of the College. All freemen of the new Company were to take an oath which had seven separate clauses.

The draft received severe criticism from all interested parties, and it was not until the preparation of second and third drafts that the charter finally passed the Great Seal on 6 December 1617. The most important changes from the first draft are to be found in the freeman's oath, which from the physicians' point of view was completely emasculated. The apothecaries were *not* confined to the formulae of the new

[9] G. Unwin, *Industrial organisation in the sixteenth and seventeenth centuries*, Oxford, Clarendon Press, 1904, p. 201.

antidotary, or to dispensing only those prescriptions written by licensees of the College. The recommendations regarding registers were dropped, as were restrictions on the supply of poisons, and, most important of all with far-reaching effects, nowhere were apothecaries forbidden to give advice or medicine either in the patient's home or in the shop. Wall and Cameron believed that Sir Francis Bacon, no lover of physicians, thus deliberately frustrated the designs of the College to make the apothecaries totally subservient to it.[10]

The position of the new Company was far from secure until at least the Civil War. It soon ran up against another newly constituted company, that of the Distillers; far from receiving support from Mayerne, they were bluntly told that the purpose of the apothecaries' charter was to make sure that they dispensed the physician's prescriptions as he required them to be done, and ". . . not abuse the powers put in their hands but content themselves to use them with order, modesty and reverence to their superiors, the physicians." In 1630, the College decided the time was ripe to tighten its hold over the apothecaries. The physicians demanded that the apothecaries should in future take an even more comprehensive oath, one which they could only interpret as an intolerable insult to their integrity. This was backed by four further demands two years later, one of which was that the College should supervise the pricing of medicines.

The apothecaries were not intimidated, and fought back with vigour. The College issued a manifesto, complaining that the apothecaries aided unlicensed physicians, but the Society replied firmly that they were freemen of the City and so entitled to trade with all, and, in any case, there were many doctors of medicine in practice both in London and the rest of England who were not members of the College. Possibly the requirement the apothecaries found most infuriating was that they should bring all their wares to the College for testing before they were put up for sale. In the end, the Company told the College bluntly that the apothecary's skill and honesty should only be subject to the control of his own organization, and, besides, the physicians were not competent to judge his wares.

The whole quarrel came to a head with the small matter of whether lac sulphuris might be sold by the apothecaries or not. The College appealed to the privy council and the attorney-general. The latter entered a "quo warranto" suit, and the privy council in 1639–40 appointed a body of referees, who seem to have been far from impartial. Their report, if accepted in full, would have deprived the Society of Apothecaries of any independent action and made it but an appendage of the College, for it included such recommendations as that the apothecaries should no longer have the right of search of their own shops except at the direction of the physicians and that their professional conduct was to be regulated by the College, from which they would receive their ordinances.[11] The Society had no alternative but to refuse to comply; happily for them, national events then overtook both parties. In the rapidly hardening divisions of the country, the king was impotent in London, and Parliament had more important things to debate.

At the Restoration, the fortunes of the College of Physicians were at low ebb and

[10] Wall, Cameron, and Underwood, op. cit., note 8 above, p. 20.
[11] Clark, op. cit., note 7 above, p. 272.

they were forced to introduce the concept of the "honorary fellow". There were many doctors in London who had good reputations as men and scholars but who were neither fellows nor candidates. The new fellows were admitted without examination and on payment of £20; as the first list of 1664 held seventy-three names, the College made a very handsome sum of money. The physicians had received their new charter from Charles II in March 1663, and were once more in a position to do battle with the apothecaries, who, in their opinion, had become thoroughly out of hand. Almost immediately, however, the Great Plague erupted, an event that did little to improve the image of the physicians in the eyes of the public.

The attacks of the physicians in their pamphlets were so virulent that one suspects they were nervous, even frightened, men. Possibly some of the more percipient feared they were waging a war which would ultimately go against them; one of them wrote in reply to *Medice, cura teipsum* (1671), "The sick call the Apothecary, Doctor; if allowed to do so they will soon think him a fit and lawful practitioner." Apparently despairing of controlling the apothecaries by earlier methods, they made a foray into the enemy's own country by establishing in June 1697 their own dispensary at Warwick Lane, to be followed by two branches. By no means all of the College's members were in agreement, and many, such as Robert Pitt (later to change his views), Tancred Robinson (friend of the apothecary, James Petiver), Hugh Chamberlen, Francis Barnard (originally an apothecary himself), and Edward Baynard (who started life as a surgeon's apprentice) refused to sign the approval for making medicines at the College.

Whether the dispensaries were just one more manoeuvre in the physicians' fight, or whether there was a genuine element of philanthropy is debatable. Perhaps both were present at first, but the endeavour to obtain a contract for the supply of drugs to the navy seems to have had little to commend it. Possibly a lucrative contract was desperately needed to ease the physicians' severe financial difficulties, and at the same time it would be denied to the apothecaries, but one inclines to the view that plain greed was the motive. In the event, the Society came well out of the business, because it gained all the later naval contracts. The tide was running strongly in the favour of the apothecaries.

In February 1701, William Rose, apothecary, was sued in the court of Queen's Bench by the College of Physicians under the Act of Henry VIII for practising physic. There was no doubt that he had been summoned to the sick man and that he had prescribed and supplied boluses, electuaries, and juleps, but the jury was unsure if this constituted practising as a physician in such a way as was prohibited by the Act – an admission of the degree to which the public had accepted the physic-practising apothecary. After protracted discussion, the court found for the College. As is well known, a reversal of decision was obtained in the House of Lords on 15 March 1704. The peers' view was that the earlier judgment was not only contrary to custom but that the advice and the treatment given by apothecaries was in the public interest. Before the Rose case, the apothecary had not charged a consultation fee, a custom which the Lords confirmed was to be continued. In future, the apothecary would have the legal right to diagnose, to advise, and to prescribe, however serious the illness, but he was not to charge for these services, only for the medical preparations supplied.[12]

8

This must have led to over-prescribing, but was not necessarily the cause of a national ineradicable demand for large quantities of physic, as is often alleged; a number of other western European countries with a totally different tradition behind them consume today considerably more "pills and potions" than England.

Puzzlement has more than once been expressed at Samuel Dodd's plea during the hearing in the House of Lords, that the reversal of the earlier finding would be to the benefit, ". . . not only for the apothecaries but for all the poor people of England." Rose's patient, John Searle, a butcher, had received a bill for £50, a large sum of money.[13] The answer lies in the statement of the apothecaries' counsel in 1694, when the Society successfully petitioned that all freemen of the Society and all provincial apothecaries who had seven-year apprenticeships behind them, should be exempt from municipal office and jury service. He had said that his clients had nineteen-twentieths of all the medical practice in London, including all that of the *sick poor* – a reference to the fact that it was the apothecary (and often the surgeon too) and not the physician who was called in by the parish Overseers of the Poor to attend their sick poor (see pp. 31ff).

During the years prior to the Rose case and immediately afterwards, two groups of people, the druggists and the "chymists", grew in number. They both dealt in apothecary wares to an extent that alarmed the Society, which, in 1721, approached the College, suggesting they should join together in the regulation of pharmacy. They did not receive the support for which they had hoped, the physicians alleging that the College and the Society already held adequate powers for dealing with the problem. Despite this answer, two years later, the College decided to promote their own Bill asking for new powers, "to search the shops of druggists and chymists and all vendors of medicines as they do now apothecaries."[14] The apothecaries petitioned against it, on the grounds that no medicine should be destroyed without the agreement of their own wardens, as the physicians were incompetent to judge faulty drugs. The Bill, however, passed, without the apothecaries' amendment, in May 1724 (10 Geo. I c. 20); the Act was limited to a period of three years.

It was renewed in 1727, in spite of further opposition by the apothecaries, who even went so far as to think of testing the physicians' expertise in the assessment of drugs. Again, the Act had a three-year limit imposed on it. When it came up for a further renewal in early 1730, the apothecaries made it known that they would only let it go forward unopposed if their wardens were granted an equal share of power. They knew they were on fairly safe ground and that their accusation of incompetence was well founded, because when James Goodwin, chemist and apothecary (though not a freeman of the Company), appealed to the whole College against the decision of the censors to burn five of his preparations, type-specimens had to be obtained from

---

[12] This clause was not rescinded until 1830 as a result of the case Handey v. Henson.

[13] Holmes, op. cit., note 2 above, p. 187. ". . . 'but for all the poor people of England' [provided, one must presume, the poor had £50 to spare]."

[14] Wall, Cameron, and Underwood, op. cit., note 8 above, p. 184. Why the Physicians should have decided on this Bill is not at all clear, as the charter granted to the College by James I laid down that the censors ". . . shall and may have full and absolute power . . . to enter into the House Shoppe Cellar Vault Workehouse or other rooms of the house of any Apothecarie Druggist Distiller and Sellers of Waters Oyles or other compositions. . . ."

Apothecaries' Hall.[15] The physicians refused to concede anything, but the Bill failed and the Act expired.

After these tests of strength, the two parties settled down to a period of peace. For the apothecaries, however, the problem of the chemists and druggists became ever more pressing. In 1724, they contemplated promoting an Act "for a General View of Medicines over England", which included arrangements for co-operation with apothecaries in other cities.[16] Though difficult to operate, this could have had desirable consequences, and, as we have just seen, was not the first time the Society had shown a concern for the provinces.[17] Two years' work was carried out on the 1724 proposal but it was then dropped, and not revived until 1746.

It is obvious from the declining numbers of the Society in 1746 that there were many apothecaries practising in London who were not members. In order to coerce them into joining, the court of assistants ordered the drafting of a Bill, "to oblige all apothecaries and other persons making and keeping medicines for sale within the limits of the Company's charter, to be examined and admitted members of this Society." Apart from bringing wayward apothecaries into the fold, chemists and druggists were to be forced to become brethren. Powers of search in all such establishments were also sought. The useless exercise of seeking the College's co-operation was not entered into; when they did show the proposed Bill to the physicians, they received the not unexpected reply that it would be opposed. Naturally, the Bill was resented by the chemists and druggists, but it was not their efforts that caused its failure. The physicians made an underground attempt to revive and make perpetual the Act of 1724, which put the apothecaries in the extraordinary position of having to fight what should have been their own Bill. Parliament was prorogued before any final decisions were made.

The failed Bill provides evidence that efforts were being made to band together the apothecaries on a national basis. After the petition from the Society, which was supported by a similar application from the non-freemen of Westminster and the City, there were in quick succession petitions from the apothecaries of Chester and Shrewsbury, in which they suggested that legislation should be extended to the rest of the country. From the examination of the witnesses, there would seem to be little doubt that it was normal practice for the chemists and druggists to send their inferior materials to country apothecaries. One witness, William (later Sir William, MD) Watson, apothecary, botanist, and experimenter in electricity, was of the opinion that two-thirds of the drugs used in the country originated in London and that the bulk of the trade was in the hands of the chemists and druggists.[18] It was rare for a London guild to have juridical powers over provincial craftsmen, two exceptions being the Framework-Knitters' Company and that of the Pewterers. Administrative problems were considerable, but the Society does not seem to have been unduly daunted.[19]

---

[15] Clark, op. cit., note 7 above, p. 495.

[16] Wall, Cameron, and Underwood, op. cit., note 8 above, p. 185.

[17] Clark, op. cit., note 7 above, pp. 442–443. The Act of 6 & 7 Wm. III c. 4 was renewed in 1702 and 1712 and made perpetual in 1722.

[18] 'Attempted legislation in 1748', *Chem. Drugg.*, 1926, **105**: 198–199.

[19] The Framework-Knitters' Company had written into its charter executive powers extending throughout England and Wales, and all mayors, bailiffs, constables, etc., were ordered to assist the officers

The inquiry into the Bill also revealed the number of shops involved. John Staples, the beadle of the Society, related that their searchers visited once a year all apothecaries' and chemists' shops, whether they belonged to freemen or to "foreigners" within the area of the Company's charter and that they amounted to some 700, at least half of which did not belong to men free of the Company. He added that the druggists' shops did not receive such visitations, and he had not included them in his figures.[20] If these figures are to be believed, the size of the problem facing the apothecaries was immense; the physicians may well have been relieved that their revived Bill of 1748 came to nought.

The first half of the eighteenth century was not a period of great activity for the physicians, and their relationship with the surgeons was even quieter than it was with the apothecaries. Dissent between physicians and surgeons nearly always hinged on the use of internal medicines, something which was forbidden to the latter. Time and again, they presented Bills and petitions to try and gain this right but were unsuccessful. After about 1706, the College paid little attention to the surgeons and we can guess that the regulation was generally flouted.[21] Relations between the Company of Barber-Surgeons and the Society of Apothecaries were, as a rule, amiable. The Society had opposed the surgeons in 1689 in the matter of internal medicines, but the two quickly came to agreement in 1705 before the presentation of the next Bill. The apothecaries had the Rose case safely behind them, and the two groups drew closer together.

The surgeons were much irked by the episcopal powers inherent in the Act of 1511, and in 1689 sought for themselves the sole examining and licensing powers for surgery. In this they were unsuccessful, but the bishops became less and less interested in wielding their power and scarcely exerted themselves after the first two decades of the eighteenth century. The surgeons had an altogether different problem then.

The Cromwellian ordinance authorizing disbanded soldiers to practise a trade to which they had not been apprenticed was re-enacted in 1660,[22] and again later. On 15 April 1709, a complaint was brought in the court of the Barber-Surgeons' Company that Henry Drudge was "exercising Barbery and Surgery within the City not being free." He "alleged that he having been a soldier in the late Warr thought himself intituled to keep his shopp without takeing up his Freedom by virtue of the Act of parliament made upon the disbanding the Army which gives liberty to disbanded soldiers to exercise any trade within the Corporations or places where they were borne although they had not served seven years to it." The court believed that they had found a loophole, as Drudge had not been born in London, and ". . . ordered that in Case he did not shut up his Shop in a Months time he should be presented upon the

---

of the Company. See R. J. Blackman, *London's livery companies*, London, Sampson Low, Marston, [n.d.], p. 202. The jurisdiction of the London Pewterers over standards of production was extended throughout the realm by virtue of their charter. See J. Hatcher and T. C. Barker, *A history of British pewter*, London, Longman, 1974, p. 174.

[20] In spite of the failure of the Act, the College continued to visit chemists and druggists until March 1856, but even when a shop was reported to be of a very poor standard, they do not seem to have tried to exact penalties. See L. Dopson, 'State of London chemists' shops in the 18th and early 19th centuries', *Chem. Drugg.*, 1955, **163**: 718–721.

[21] Clark, op. cit. note 7 above, p. 500.

[22] C. Hill, *The century of revolution, 1630–1714*, Walton-on-Thames, Thomas Nelson, 1980, p. 176.

11

statute made in the 32nd. year of King Henry VIII."[23] Nothing more seems to be recorded of the matter.

The Surgeons' Company, after its separation from the barbers of the old Barber-Surgeons' Company, had even less coercive powers than their predecessor, owing to the loose manner in which their constitution had been drawn up. In 1749, an Act was passed that allowed, "such officers, marines and soldiers as have been in his Majesty's service since the accession of George II to set up in trade without any let, suit or molestation", even though they had served no apprenticeship. The new Company was in no position to enforce the examination of such men who practised as surgeons, nor could they exact any penalty, which unfortunate situation was fully confirmed by Sir Dudley Ryder.[24] In 1763, another Act extended the exemption to those who had been in the services since 1749, and went so far as to include their wives and children as well. Counsels' opinions were again sought, but their views were no more encouraging.

Thus, even in London, by the mid-eighteenth century, the neat boundaries and spheres of influence of the sixteenth and seventeenth centuries beloved of many medical historians had faded away.[25] The physicians had failed to control the apothecaries, the apothecaries gave up all attempts to control the chemists and druggists, and the surgeons were quite unable to control the retired army and navy surgeons.

The position in the provinces was even more fluid. Raach has shown that between 1603 and 1643 there were 800 physicians outside London, almost ten times the number admitted by the College for practice inside London and thirty-two times greater than the extra-licentiates; three-quarters of them had matriculated, and a quarter had an MD, but, as Roberts noted, Raach's *Directory* gives no hint that many of the physicians listed were in fact surgeons and apothecaries practising physic who had taken out episcopal licences.[26] Nor is this surprising, for the case of Thomas Edwards, apothecary of Exeter, in 1607, in which he won the right to practise as a physician was as great a watershed in the provinces as the Rose case in London a hundred years later.

The licences granted by the episcopal authorities had little to do with a man's medical qualifications, indeed, they were usually issued *after* he had been in practice for years; as Rowse wrote, they were rather "certificates of honesty and good conduct".[27] The College made a feeble attempt in 1556 to control provincial practice, and a few prosecutions took place, but we must suppose that any other control that was exerted must have lain with the guilds, to which, by an Act of Edward III in 1363, every man practising a trade had to belong.

No town outside the capital was large enough to possess single, unmixed guilds for

[23] Guildhall Library, Company of Barber-Surgeons' court minutes, MS. 5257/7, f. 31.

[24] C. Wall, *The history of the Surgeons' Company, 1745–1800*, London, Hutchinson, 1937, p. 139.

[25] Wall, Cameron, and Underwood, op. cit., note 8 above, p. 188. Writing of a period as late as the 1770s, they stated: "The healing art was still looked upon as divided into separate territories presided over by different corporations and none must encroach upon the other. The surgeons ruled their own domain and no apothecary must venture to conduct the most trivial surgical procedure."

[26] R. S. Roberts, 'The personnel and practice of medicine in Tudor and Stuart England', Part I: 'The provinces', *Med. Hist.*, 1962, **6**: 363–382, see p. 363.

[27] A. L. Rowse, *The Elizabethan renaissance, the cultural achievement*, London, Macmillan, 1972, p. 260.

either the barber-surgeons or the apothecaries. Matthews successfully traced the line of descent of those who dealt in apothecary wares and pharmacy from the spicer of the thirteenth century to the grocer of the fifteenth and the apothecary of the next century in the towns of York, Leicester, Norwich, and Canterbury.[28] In Canterbury, the apothecaries were in a fellowship that included grocers, chandlers, and fishmongers; in Leicester, they were in a large guild of merchants, whilst in Norwich they were, in 1561, associated with physicians and barber-surgeons, but, after civic re-organization in 1622, they were placed in the fourth company, which comprised upholders, tanners, and others. The Fraternity of the Blessed Mary in York became, in 1408, the Guild of Corpus Christi, which, in its turn, was incorporated in 1581 into the wealthy Merchant Adventurers' Company, which included apothecaries, mercers, grocers, and ironmongers.[29]

The boundaries between the different guilds were by no means hard and fast. Berger has shown that a protracted battle went on between the Barber-Surgeons' and the Mercers' companies of Coventry for the allegiance of the apothecaries. In 1578, the former prosecuted a non-freeman before the mayor and council for illegally retailing drugs, yet in 1593, the latter, while ratifying a new set of by-laws, claimed that the town's apothecaries were under their control.[30] Berger believes them to have been evenly divided between the two groups.

There is no reason to suppose that the provincial guilds were any more vigorous than their London contemporaries in pursuing errant freemen and non-freemen, but records are, on the whole, scant. Where they do exist, as, for example, those of the Barber-Surgeons' and Tallow-Chandlers' Company and the Mercers', Grocers' Apothecaries' and Ironmongers' Company of Chester, the records deteriorate so rapidly and so completely after about 1720 that it seems reasonable to suppose that there had been a collapse in guild power. A similar picture is to be seen at Bristol, except that the date was some thirty years later.[31]

It should not be forgotten in considering the organization of medical practice in the provinces that by no means all towns had guilds; indeed, in 1689, of 200 towns in England, only a quarter had any organized guilds at all.[32] It is frequently stated, and probably with much truth, that the prosperity of the rapidly rising industrial towns such as Birmingham was due to the fact that they were not chartered boroughs, had no guilds, and Dissenters were free from the restrictions imposed by the Clarendon Code. The practice of medicine and pharmacy must have been equally free from control, though with what result is not always clear.

[28] L. G. Matthews, 'Spicers and apothecaries in the city of Canterbury', *Med. Hist.*, 1965, **9**: 289–291; *idem*, 'The spicers and apothecaries of Norwich', *Pharm. J.*, 1967, **198**: 5–9; *idem*, 'The city of York's first spicers, grocers and apothecaries', *Pharm. Hist.*, 1971, **1**: pt 1, 2–3.

[29] For Norwich, see Margaret Pelling and Charles Webster, 'Medical practitioners', in C. Webster (editor), *Health, medicine and mortality in the sixteenth century*, Cambridge University Press, 1979, pp. 165–235, see pp. 210–215; and Margaret Pelling's paper in *Scienze, credenze occulte, livelli di cultura*, Florence, Olschki, 1982. For York, see T. D. Whittet, 'The apothecary in provincial gilds', *Med. Hist.*, 1964, **8**: 245–273, see p. 259.

[30] R. M. Berger, 'Mercantile careers in the early seventeenth century: Thomas Atherall, a Coventry apothecary', *Warks. Hist.*, 1981–2, **5**: 37–51, see p. 42.

[31] For a fuller discussion, see J. Burnby, 'Apprenticeship records', *Trans. Br. Soc. Hist. Pharm.*, 1977, **1**: 145–177, see pp. 172–174.

[32] Hill, op. cit., note 22 above, p. 176.

II

JOB DESCRIPTION

The modern concept of "job descriptions" with the legal protection of professional titles did not develop until the second half of the nineteenth century. Today, the dividing lines are so finely drawn that, not only do we differentiate between butcher, baker, and candlestick-maker, but between structural and civil engineers, systems and stress analysts, clinicians, clinical pharmacologists and clinical pharmacists, haematologists, gynaecologists and neurologists, and so on. So imbued are we with these ideas and their importance to us, that it is difficult to relate to a different outlook. The charters of the City of London's many companies do not help us in this readjustment.

The Gardeners' Company was established in 1606, its authority extending to a six-mile radius around the City, within which area it was to control, "the trade, crafte or misterie of gardening, planting, grafting, setting, sowing, cutting, arboring . . . fencing and removing of plantes, herbes, seedes, fruites, trees. . . ." It was empowered to search for and destroy any unwholesome or rotten goods in the markets, and no one could set up as a gardener without permission, that is, membership was obligatory. In practice, this was not the case. John Noble of Hoxton, a well-known and successful horticulturalist of the first half of the seventeenth century, was a member of the Tallow-Chandlers' Company. He had at least eight apprentices, four of whom were admitted to the freedom of the Tallow-Chandlers; they, in their turn, had apprentices, so that in the course of time there grew up a fair number of gardeners within the body of the Company of Tallow-Chandlers.[33] The records of the company do not indicate that these men were gardeners; that information comes from other sources. Thomas Fairchild, also of Hoxton, a gardener of greater fame, was a member of the Worshipful Company of Clothworkers. The chemist George Wilson (1631–1711), as his will attests, was a citizen and haberdasher.[34] There was no company specially formed for the needs of "chymists", and so the Haberdashers' Company was presumably as good as any other to Wilson, but one wonders why John Cluer and William Dicey, printers and at a later date patent medicine vendors, chose the Leathersellers' Company in preference to the Stationers.[35]

There were few societies as meticulous in their records as the Society of Friends, who went to some trouble to secure precision. When, on 23 October 1735, John Sherwin married Mercy Oakey, the scribe was careful to state that John was a "citizen and draper of London, by trade a baker".[36] Likewise, when John Bell of Lombard Street married Elizabeth Foggs in September 1710, he was described as "A hozier but by company citizen and bowstring maker". Sixty years later, his great-

---

[33] Guildhall Library, Company of Tallow-Chandlers' presentations, MSS. 6152/2 and 3.

[34] He obtained his freedom 27 November 1668 by order of the Court of Aldermen.

[35] The Leathersellers' Company Freedoms' Register, "William Dicey, Apprentice of John Sewers by Indenture dated 17 April 1711, he having been turned over to John Cluer, Stationer. Obtained the Freedom on 7th August, 1721."

[36] Friends' Library, accumulated records for London and Middlesex, marriages.

nephew (father of John Bell, chemist and druggist), Jacob Bell of Fish Street Hill, was described in similar terms.

No company was more mixed than that of the Barber-Surgeons. For a period after 1635, in the freedom records the master's trade is frequently given. The term barber-surgeon was scarcely used, but rather barber or chirurgeon, but what is very noticeable are the numbers of dyers, innkeepers, distillers, and hosiers, as well as a few box-makers, sheargrinders, grocers, button-makers, wheelwrights, cutlers, upholsterers, and even a gun-maker. There were, at one time, two Peter Watts, one a wire-drawer and the other a carpenter, but their careers are impossible to sort out, as on other occasions they are simply termed citizen and barber-surgeon.

Translation from one company to another was common. "5 April 1709. Sherrington Somerfeild summon'd for keeping a barbers shop not being free of this Company, came and alleg'd that he served his time to a barber free of the Company of Haberdashers and was himself free of that Company whereupon the Court gave him time till the first Tuesday in July to take up his Freedom of this Company at three guineas."[37] A problem is posed by the following type of entry: "7 October 1733. Ed. Ledger who was apprentice of William Serles, Barber, and afterwards of Anthony Bayles, Haberdasher was admitted into the Freedom by Service upon Testimony of said Anthony Bayles."[37a] But was he a barber or a haberdasher?

Holmes, in his study of the medical profession, makes reference to the "bargain-basement" for apprenticeship premiums. "There were a great many barber-surgeons after 1700, in London as well as in the provinces, who still took on apprentices for five, six or seven years at a minimal charge – for anything from £12 down to £5, in fact. It can be safely assumed that they dispensed little in the way of a genuine medical training. . . ."[38] In fact, it cannot be assumed, particularly in London, that these lowly-priced apprentice-masters, described as citizens and barber-surgeons, were barber-surgeons at all; they were just as likely, probably more likely, to have been hosiers or cordwainers.

The problem is undoubtedly as great in the provinces, but even more difficult to detect. Only London, by far the largest town in England throughout its history, was big enough to support sufficient individual companies to cover the activities of most occupations. In the provinces, it was necessary to group trades together, often apparently in a completely arbitrary fashion, such as the barber-surgeons with the silk-weavers in Salisbury. The apothecaries, on the other hand, were in a Merchants' Company, re-named the Grocers' Company in 1613, which comprised grocers, mercers, goldsmiths, linen-drapers, milliners, vintners, upholsterers, and embroiderers.[39] In many towns, the wealthiest men were the mercers, and it was their title that came first in any composite guild, for example, the Mercers, Ironmongers, Grocers and Apothecaries of Chester, or, as at Lichfield, where an all-embracing guild was simply known as the Mercers' Guild. This could lead to confusion in the description adopted by a trader.

---

[37] Guildhall Library, Barber-Surgeons' Company's court minutes, MS. 5257/7, f. 30.
[37a] Ibid., Barber-Surgeons' Company's Freedoms, MS. 5265/5, f. 8.
[38] Holmes, op. cit., note 2 above, p. 216.
[39] C. Haskins, *Ancient trade guilds and companies of Salisbury*, Salisbury, Bennett, 1912, pp. 80, 364.

Whittet has related how Robert Blease, apprentice of Adam Blease, mercer and apothecary, a councillor of Chester in 1582, is sometimes described in the records as mercer and in others as apothecary.[40] John Palmer senior of Coventry, when taking an apprentice in 1722, called himself mercer and apothecary, but although in the Middle Ages mercers dealt in spices and drugs, there is no reason to believe that the two occupations were connected in the eighteenth century. The explanation is that many apothecaries in Coventry were members of the Mercers' Company.[41] This may well be the explanation why on trade tokens a man's stated occupation on one side varies from the company's arms on the other, as noted by Trease.[42]

A man's true title of occupation having been determined, the difficult problem of his job description then arises. This is of particular importance in any discussion of the English apothecary, owing to the unusual manner in which his "art and mystery" has developed in this country.

The most general belief is that in the medieval period he was a preparer and purveyor of drugs, and did not prescribe or directly participate in the patient's treatment, but by the late seventeenth century had wandered increasingly into the attractive fields of medical practice, something that was given legal sanction with the Rose case of 1703; by the end of that century and the Apothecaries' Act of 1815, he was recognized to be a doctor. D'Arcy Power and Rolleston have claimed that the medieval apothecary, besides being a seller of simples and preparer of compounds, was also a prescriber and medical attendant.[43] This view has often been challenged, but some support for it can be found in an inquiry held on 28 February 1354. On that day, the Prior of Hogges, Master Paschel, Master Adams de la Poletrie, and Master David de Westmerland, surgeons, were put on oath to determine whether John le Spicer de Cornhulle had been guilty of negligence in treating a wound of Thomas de Shene.[44] Trease has shown that the terms spicer and apothecary were virtually interchangeable, but what is particularly noticeable is that the spicer's right to give treatment was not being challenged, but only that he had been negligent.

Some eighty years later, in 1433, an interesting case occurred in the city of York. The prior of Guisborough and one of his canons, Brother Richard Ayreton, demanded £40 damages from Matthew Rillesford, leech of York, for malpractice in the treatment of Richard's leg. On 14 September, the three men put the two sides of the case before Robert Belton of York, apothecary. Belton's decision was that during the following eight days Rillesford was to apply his treatment to Brother Richard's leg under Belton's own supervision, and that the clerics were to drop their action against

[40] Whittet, op. cit., note 29 above, p. 258.

[41] Public Record Office (PRO), Inland Revenue apprenticeship records, I.R./1/48 f. 18. Berger has shown that the apothecaries in Coventry were split between the Mercers' and the Barber-Surgeons' companies, see op. cit., note 30 above, p. 42. See also, Joan Lane, *Coventry apprentices and their masters 1781–1806*, Stratford-upon-Avon, Dugdale Society, 1983.

[42] G. E. Trease, *Pharmacy in history*, London, Baillière, Tindall & Cox, 1964, pp. 145, 128. He also refers to Ralph Clark being termed a mercer, but that his inventory of 1631 shows clearly that he was an apothecary.

[43] D'Arcy Power, 'English medicine and surgery in the fourteenth century', *Selected writings, 1877–1930*, Oxford, Clarendon Press, 1931, p. 43; H. Rolleston, 'History of medicine in the city of London', *Ann. med. Hist.*, 1941, **3**: 3. Both cite the case of Coursus de Gangeland.

[44] R. R. Sharpe (editor), *Calendar of the letter books . . . of the archives of the city of London*, 1889–1912, Letter book G, p. 21.

the leech for negligence before 14 September. The plaintiffs were not satisfied with this decision and the case went before a jury.[45] The final outcome is not known but the main interest lies in the fact that an apothecary was regarded as being of sufficient status and of sufficient medical experience to arbitrate in a case of alleged medical incompetence.

Roberts, making use of a famous passage of arms between John Woolton MD (Oxon), son of a former bishop, and Thomas Edwards, apothecary of Exeter, has shown that apothecaries were practising medicine in that city from at least the 1590s – and very successfully too.[46] Rook and Newbold, on the basis of a detailed analysis of the medical scene in Cambridge from 1558 to 1642, came to a similar conclusion. They wrote: "... the rigid tripartite division of medical activities described by so many historians, though it may well have prevailed in London, was not a conspicuous feature of medical life in Cambridge.... It is apparent that in the sixteenth and seventeenth centuries almost all medical men whether they were by training physicians, surgeons, or apothecaries, were in effect general practitioners. It may have been true, as was apparently the case in London, that the richer patients tended in the first instance to consult a physician and the poor an apothecary, but even this is questionable since many of the apothecaries were men of great reputation."[47]

The situation in London may well not have been so very different from that in Exeter and Cambridge. In the battle between the College of Physicians and the Society of Apothecaries, which came to a head in 1634 with a "quo warranto", the former listed a number of grievances. The third one accused the apothecaries of practising medicine, and specifically named John Buggs, George Haughton, and Richard Edwards. There is no doubt that such well-known men as John Reeve, apothecary and medical adviser to the Earl of Exeter, Thomas Johnson, the botanist, and the detested Nicholas Culpeper all practised medicine.[48] The apothecaries made their point during the Great Plague of 1665 that in future they had to be accepted as doctors, though there is little doubt that they were already well established, otherwise it is difficult to see why Nathaniel Upton, apothecary, should have been appointed master of the City pesthouse in Finsbury Fields. That there were before 1665 two types of London apothecary is made clear by William Boghurst, the apothecary, who did such yeoman service during the epidemic. He wrote, "But those apothecaries which have their work and dependence from the physitian are not, I think, obliged to stay behind when their Masters lead the way: for who shall direct them? They say it is not our business to direct or undertake to give Physick of our own heads; therefore they are to be excused. But those Apothecaries which stand upon their own legs, and live by their own practice, are bound by their undertakings to stay and help as in other diseases."[49]

[45] W. Baildon, 'Notes on the religious and secular houses of Yorkshire', *Yorks. Arch. Soc. Rec.*, 1895, **17**: 78. The leech's denial of negligence makes it plain that internal medicines had been administered.

[46] Roberts, op. cit., note 26 above, pp. 371–374.

[47] A. Rook and M. Newbold, 'Physicians, surgeons and apothecaries in Elizabethan and Stuart Cambridge', unpublished paper read before the British Society for the History of Pharmacy Conference at Cambridge in 1974.

[48] Wall, Cameron, and Underwood, op. cit., note 8 above, vol. 1, pp. 283, 301, 43, 44.

[49] T. D. Whittet, *The apothecaries in the Great Plague of London, 1665*, Epsom, A. E. Morgan Publications, 1965, pp. 24, 21.

Wall has written, "It is clear from literature of the period that the ordinary surgeon could not make a living if he confined his activities to the treatment of external diseases and accidents. He was compelled to keep a shop and to sell drugs, and to practise midwifery...."[50] James Yonge wrote in his *Journal* in 1693, "The beginning of this year I had prepared to send my son John to Leyden to travel and study", but when John's secret marriage had been discovered, James had "... stopt his voyage to Holland and put them to live at the dock, furnisht his shop, gave him some money and all the profit of the place, which was a good £100, besides practice."[51] Others had different sidelines, such as Robert Murrell of Enfield, who leased the Greyhound inn and owned a small brewery, as did his successor Joseph Wilson.

Apothecaries and surgeon/apothecaries were in the same situation. John Fage (d. 1694), apothecary of Cambridge, was also a vintner. William Fuller, surgeon and apothecary of Hemel Hempstead, established the Bell in Market Street, where he brewed his own beer and cider, and his inventory of 1671 shows he sold, "Raisins, currans, salt, starch and all other Grocery commodities".[52] There were, of course, such well-known figures as William Cookworthy, the originator and manufacturer of English porcelain; or the master of George Crabbe, John Page of Wickhambrook, Suffolk, more farmer than apothecary.[53] Each of them had an open shop, and the point of interest is, how much of an apothecary's income was derived from it, and how much from medical practice?

Trease has shown that inventories can be used to determine what groceries, sweetmeats, or drugs they sold in their shops, what apparatus they had, the size of their houses, and the value of their furnishings and apparel. Richard Beresford of Lincoln (1607) was appraised at £295; amongst his tobacco, packthread, and groceries, there was a brass syringe, five glister-pipes and urinals, which suggest that he administered enemas.[54] Samuel Newboult, a Lichfield apothecary, left a much more modest estate, a mere £74, of which the shop and the sweetmeats accounted for £33. There is no suggestion that Newboult was a medical practitioner, and the same applies to John Parker of the same city (1655). Parker's trade goods amounted to £182 (of which "Grocery, tobacco, allam, oyle etc." in the cellar was by far the largest item), a high proportion of the total of £228.[55] A similar balance can be seen in the case of Thomas Needham of Chesterfield (1665), his household goods being worth £45 and

[50] Wall, op. cit., note 24 above, p. 90.

[51] F. N. L. Poynter (editor), *The journal of James Yonge, 1647–1721*, London, Longmans, 1963, p. 205.

[52] T. D. Whittet and M. Newbold, 'Apothecaries in the diary of Samuel Newton, alderman of Cambridge', *Pharm. J.*, 1978, **221**: 118. The rating lists of Great St Mary's show that he became the occupier of the Rose inn in 1679; A. L. Wood, 'Hemel Hempstead and its people during the seventeenth and eighteenth centuries', in Susan Yaxley (editor), *History of Hemel Hempstead*, Borough of Hemel Hempstead, 1973, pp. 80–81.

[53] George Crabbe's father paid £70 to John Smith for the privilege of this doubtful apprenticeship for his son. After two years, he was removed and bound to John Page of Woodbridge for four years, the premium being only £10 on this occasion. See PRO, I.R./1/57, f. 5 and I.R./1/58, f. 9.

[54] Trease, op. cit., note 42 above, p. 127. The administration of enemas was a recognized part of the apothecary's practice, see *The gentleman apothecary: being a late and true story turned out of French*, London, [for H. Brome], 1670.

[55] D. G. Vaisey (editor), 'Probate inventories of Lichfield and district, 1568–1680', *Collections for a history of Staffordshire*, 4th ser., 1969, vol. 5, pp. 156–161, 99–102. It should be noted, however, that Parker's inventory was not completed and he is known to have leased furniture with his house.

those of the shop £120. Besides two stills, a three-bit gimblet, crucibles, and a press for oil, he had also leeches, lancets, urinals, fifty-one glister pipes, and breast glasses, which seems to indicate small-time manufacturing and medical practice.[56]

Although the sums of money for some apothecaries were low, for example, Henry Mawe of Epworth (1677) and Richard Cotterall of Alford (1679) with £31 and £63 respectively, the general impression is that most apothecaries were comfortably placed. Indeed, some could be described as wealthy. The inventory of John Inkersall of Boston (1684) came to £1,140, and that of William Franceys of Derby (1703) to nearly £800, his drugs alone amounting to £300.[57] Like other wealthy tradesmen and merchants of the period, as banking was still in its infancy, apothecaries often acted as financial middlemen. By the post-Restoration period, merchants had become familiar with the use of bills of exchange and used them for raising money. Some who wished to lend money for a short period would even buy them, but if the transactions did not proceed smoothly, then great difficulty might be experienced in recovering the cash. A safer vehicle, and one which was for the longer period of six months to a year, was the bond; in this case the penalties against the defaulters were more severe and far more enforceable. After the 1640s, mortgages became commoner, as the penalty of immediate foreclosure was no longer invoked if the defaulter could prove that he could make regular and sizeable interest payments.[58]

The goods in the shop of the Bristol apothecary, Richard Kerwood, in 1693 amounted to £5 out of his estate of £316. He had £101 in ready money but the next biggest item was, "One mortgage of a house in Ballance Streete in Bristoll of one John Tugwell – £70." There was also the matter of a "Debt due by Mr Danyell Phillips by bond – £12."[59] William Bossley of Bakewell, Derbyshire, was even more involved in financial transactions. The appraisers in 1714 placed his total estate at £396, of which £80 was accounted for by, "In the shop: Counters boxes bottles potts druggs and all materials for or belonging to his trade there or elsewhere." The money he had out on loan either upon bond or note was considerably more, being £209 in sums varying from £9 to £120. His successor in the town, John Denman, although not so rich (he was worth £188 15s.), still had £80 in "Money due upon Bonds and Book Debts" as compared with £60 for drugs and equipment in the shop.[60] From where this money originated is but rarely indicated, possibly it was from a trade surplus, or possibly it was money deposited with them. The appraisers usually grouped all debts together, using some phrase such as "Debts due and oweing both sperate and desperate".

Philip George has made effective use of the inventory of Henry Hayes of Wisbech, who died 1702, and the well-thumbed 1721 pharmacopoeia of Jeremy Cliff of

[56] Lichfield Record Office, Thomas Needham, inventory, 1666.

[57] Trease, op. cit., note 42 above, pp. 126–128, 143; Lichfield Record Office, William Franceys, will and inventory, 1703.

[58] C. Wilson, *England's apprenticeship, 1603–1763*, London, Longman, 1971, pp. 209, 155. Wilson stated that these early bankers were recruited from a number of trades and professions, the commonest being the scriveners and goldsmiths, but Trease remarked that he and others have noted that it was not unusual for apothecaries to undertake banking. He cited the case of the substantial loans made by Richard and Edward Wood of Chesterfield. Richard (apprentice-master of Thomas Needham) must have been a man of substance, as he bought Dickfield Bridge smelting mill in 1655 for £1,100. See G. E. Trease, 'Manufacture of apothecaries' tokens', *Pharm. J.*, 1966, **197**: 324.

[59] Bristol Archives Offices, Richard Kerwood, inventory, 1693.

[60] Lichfield Record Office: William Bossley, inventory, 1693; John Denman, inventory, 1753.

Tenterden. He came to the conclusion that Cliff, in contrast to Hayes, made even the most complicated preparations. His annotated pharmacopoeia indicates that he prepared at least eighty-seven out of the possible 464 preparations, including theriac. andromach. and theriac. lond., but that the emphasis was on simple ointments, plasters, electuaries, waters, and distilled spirits. On the other hand, George estimated from Hayes's inventory that it would have been impossible for him to have compounded the more complex recipes, although he made unguenta, emplastra, electuaries, emetics, opiates, and treacle water. Hayes also made considerable use of chemical drugs, which seem to have been almost completely absent from Cliff's armamentarium.[61] To what extent the surgeons and apothecaries made their own preparations is impossible to decide. They may have had busy laboratories, or they may have bought from firms of druggists such as Estwick and Conygesby in West Smithfield, or from other apothecaries, as several did from Thomas Bott of Coventry, or directly from the London Society of Apothecaries.

In order to define more exactly the apothecary's practice, his account books, business letters, and ledgers are required, but few have survived. The day book for 1706 and 1707 of an unnamed Shrewsbury apothecary recording the cash received for goods sold over the counter or in payment of an account, gives us an idea of his business. It is apparent that he had a very brisk counter-prescribing practice, in which he sold gargles, draughts, mixtures, lohochs, ointments, and other preparations. He sold patent medicines such as "scots pills" (9*d*. a box) and "sylverlocks pills" (eight for 4*d*.), oils both volatile and fixed, gums and resins, cochineal, isinglass, spermaceti, and musk. He had a ready sale for spices, soap, and oil of lavender, as well as sago, an invalid food. He carried out phlebotomies, which varied in price from 6*d*. to 2*s*. 6*d*. There were regular entries for chemicals, for example, saltpetre, arsenic, borax, vitriol, white and red lead, and for the metals gold and silver, sold by the leaf or the shell. The sale of pigments was important to him; ivory black, vermilion, carmine, lake, umber, and Dutch pink, together with brushes, crucibles, varnish, and pencils, all figured in the records.[62] On the evidence of the cash book, the Shrewsbury apothecary sold à fair range of goods, was a busy counter-prescriber, and performed phlebotomies, but it does not give any information as to whether he dispensed physicians' prescriptions, or left his shop to make domiciliaries, either alone or in the company of a physician.

Thomas Bott of Coventry has left us rather more information. His records run from 1711 to 1734 and consist of a day book and an account book. He was by no means a cash chemist and had a large number of account customers and patients who could run up horrifying bills.[63] Each day in the day book he listed the articles supplied to each customer and gathered them together under the debtor's name in the account book. When the account was settled, it was boldly crossed through, and another

---

[61] P. George, 'A Wisbech chyrurgion', *Chem. Drugg.*, 1955, **163**: 713–715; *idem*, 'Jeremy Cliff', ibid., 1954, **162**: 211–213. George tried to make a comparison between the practices of a provincial surgeon (Hayes) and an apothecary (Cliff), but it is very likely that both men were, as was usual at that period, surgeons and apothecaries; certainly this title was used by Jeremiah Cliff when taking an apprentice in 1736.

[62] 'An apothecary's cash book', *M. & B. Pharm. Bull.*, 1956, **5**: 90–94.

[63] Derbyshire Record Office, Gresley MSS., D. 77/Bott. Lord Craven ran up a bill of £69 12*s*. 1¼*d*., a figure which, however, fades into insignificance when it is noted that Bott presented to the executors of Lady Dugdale (his half-sister) a bill for over £134.

started a few pages further on – simple but effective book-keeping.

Bott supplied a greater quantity of groceries than did the Shrewsbury man, "currans", raisins, starch, coffee, candied orange and lemon, jam, and Naples biscuits figure largely in his accounts. He sold spices, and the household of the Rt Hon. William Bromley Esq., was in receipt of large quantities of dried herbs. Medicines played an important part, particularly electuaries, vomits, purges, drops, and enemas; occasionally in the day book the whole formula is given, as with Mr Grove's bolus and potion. There is no doubt that Bott practised surgery. The day book records for 26 November 1733, "Mr Waren. Curing yr: Hand Head and attendance", and the account book shows that the charge was 5s. The cost of drawing a tooth was 12d., and a phlebotomy could be had for the same sum. Lord Craven's leg required considerable treatment. Bott made frequent visits to Craven's seat at Comb, even on occasion staying the night. For these he did not charge, leaving them all "at pleasure".

At the end of the account book Thomas Bott wrote the names and addresses of his druggist suppliers in London, and it can also be seen that he acted in a small way as a wholesaler to other apothecaries. His accountancy is not always entirely clear. It seems strange that he should have supplied Mr Bromley of Baginton with quires of writing paper, or six pigeons in August (12d.) and twelve herrings the following November (6d.); and stranger still that Mr Denham should be charged 2s. for the making of a bed gown and another 2s. for a blue damask gown. Every detail was noted. Bott's asses, presumably kept for their milk, cost him a shilling a week, at Ned Stafford's, and his mare, necessary for visiting Lord Craven and other patients, went into Mr Hall's grounds from Lammas 1731 to the following Michaelmas for 10s. The misfortune of having to pay 12d. for a trespass, and even more to the chamberlain (constable) and pinlock (keeper of the pinfold), probably decided him to move the mare to a more expensive but safer place.

Geographically, his practice covered a surprisingly wide area. He supplied or treated people as far away as Kenilworth and Stoneleigh, Atherstone, Griff, and Dunchurch; farthest away of all were Rowland Berkeley Esq., in Worcestershire, and his relations, the Armesteads, in Yorkshire. The impression is gained from these account books that Thomas Bott had a busy shop with a wide range of groceries and drugs, and a flourishing medical practice as well.

Not far away at Stafford was the apothecaries' practice of Thomas and Lewis Dickenson, father and son, for which we have account books dating from 1707–22 and 1736–55.[64] Thomas Dickenson's accounts show that, like Thomas Bott, he had a large number of account customers, although bills do not seem to have been allowed to run on for such long periods. He supplied the usual confections, juleps, draughts, and electuaries, as well as olive oil, huge quantities of manna, cream of tartar, smelling salts, and cinnamon water. His groceries were very much less, mostly tea, coffee, sago, and sugar candy, also saltpetre, bay salt, and sal prunella, probably used as food preservatives. His medical practice was busy; he bled patients, dressed their arms, prescribed "two plaisters for Mrs Hicks's breasts", and charged Benjamin Cotton 2s. 6d. for "Dressings for Sally's leg and making an issue". He applied fomentations and

[64] William Salt Library, Stafford, Hand-Morgan collection, H.M. 27/3 and 4. At one time, it was believed that the two account books belonged to one man, but it has now been established that the earlier belonged to Thomas and the later to Lewis, his son.

administered enemas, for which he charged 1*s*. 6*d*., but also supplied "arm'd pipes", presumably for self or home administration, a view supported by the frequent entries for "Ingred. pro Enem. 6*d*.".

The account book of Lewis Dickenson does not greatly differ. He still supplied treacle water and diacodium, boxes of pills, aethiops mineral, opodeldoc, and mixtures "for a Glyster". Groceries were, however, noticeably less, primarily sago and barley sugar. Lewis had a younger brother, Thomas, who was a grocer in Worcester, and it is interesting to compare his account book of 1740–50 with that of the apothecary. Thomas sold, as would be expected, several varieties of tea, coffee, cocoa, sugar, and chocolate. From letters sent to him, one learns that he was regarded as a good judge of hops; tobacco, raisins, currants, almonds, jam, candied lemon, pepper, cloves, treacle, soap, nuts, and starch all figure in his accounts, but the only true pharmaceutical products were brimstone and ague powders. As far as the two Dickenson brothers were concerned, the split between apothecary and grocer was complete.

The later day book of Maximilian Grindon of Olney (died 1784) and the accounts ledger of his son George, who practised into the nineteenth century, have a completely medical bias, unless the sale of three lemons and twelve grains of cochineal in 1789 can be regarded as evidence of a lingering interest in the sale of groceries. The two doctors sold their patients blisters, pills, balsams, and mixtures, and simple druggist lines such as creta praecip. and Glauber's salts; they also charged up to 2*s*. 6*d*. for a journey.[65] It seems that by the last quarter of the eighteenth century, the provincial apothecary had divorced himself from the sale of household commodities, whether for the bathroom, kitchen, or first-aid cupboard. He was still a dispenser of medicines, but of those prescribed by himself. He charged for his journeys if not his advice, and also sold chemist's sundries such as glister pipes and dressings. In some cases, he still had an "open shop" with heavy counter-prescribing and a ready sale in "own lines".[66] His medical practice was mixed and comprised that of surgeon, physician, and midwife.

There is also the man whom Holmes dubbed the "'pothecary-physician".[67] The phenomenon of the apothecary-turned-physician who proved his respectability by brandishing some fairly easily-won MD, is well known. The reasons for the transformation are not far to seek. It was not only a matter of status, and it is likely that the monetary returns were little better, but quite simply an easier and pleasanter life, especially for a man of advancing years. When Henry Nunn, surgeon and apothecary, and William Silk, apothecary (in later indentures called surgeon and apothecary), both of Manningtree, drew up an agreement that they were to become co-partners and ". . . joint dealers in the profession, art and business of a surgeon and apothecary in buying and selling all sorts of Drugs and Medicines necessary and incident to the Business and in administring the same and in giving advice to patients", certain conditions were written in. One was ". . . that William Silk shall at all times . . . take upon

[65] Cowper Museum, Olney, Grindon MSS. George, and probably his father too, were doctors to the poor of the parishes of Emberton and Yardley.

[66] As late as 1832–8, William Sturton LSA owned the shop alongside his home and surgery at Greenwich in which he employed his druggist brothers. The unpublished Sturton letters, copies of which are in the writer's possession.

[67] Holmes, op. cit., note 2 above, p. 204.

himself the active and laborious parts of the partnership and more particularly the apothecary's part of the business, and that Henry Nunn shall from time to time as often as he thinks proper absent himself from and shall give such attendance and application only as shall be agreeable and convenient to him."[68] In other words, Henry Nunn had decided to "take it easier", and this is just what some 'pothecary-physicians did.

Becoming a physician meant one could be more selective, but not necessarily that all future practice in surgery and pharmacy was eschewed. It is not known with any exactitude what comprised the medical practice of a newly elevated physician. Edward Spry, when he took an apprentice in 1756, called himself an apothecary, but subsequently, on gaining his Aberdeen MD, he understandably used the title "practitioner in physic". With his contemporary and neighbour, John Mudge, it was quite otherwise. He did not receive his Aberdeen MD until 1784, but he had already given himself the title of physician in 1767 when signing the indentures of William Cookworthy, and three years earlier still, that of "practitioner in physic" when becoming the master of Bartholomew Dunsterville. It would be interesting to know at what date Mudge charged substantial fees for diagnosis and advice alone, and if his general practice and shopkeeping ceased.

From data such as these, it is clear that, despite the general tendency of the apothecary to acquire more specifically medical functions during the course of the eighteenth century, caution must be exercised in the acceptance of glib titles and the over-simplification of the convenient categories used to describe medical practitioners and their practices in earlier times.

[68] Essex Record Office, MS. D/DHW B. 10.

III

THE APOTHECARY AS PROGENITOR

INTRODUCTION

In comparison with the physician, the apothecary was a practical man, though also touched by the Scientific Revolution of the late seventeenth century. Many, if not all, the roots of the ever-finer divisions of medicine, science, and pharmacy can be detected in the fertile soil of apothecarial practice. It is not too much to claim that the apothecaries of the period under discussion were amongst the precursors of the dispensing chemist, the experimental and manufacturing chemist, the pharmaceutical wholesaler and manufacturer, and the general practitioner.

As a founding father, he was by no means equally responsible for all his descendants, nor did he exert equal influence on them all. His effect on the experimental chemist was comparatively slight, neither was he pre-eminent in the rise of the manufacture of inorganic chemicals. Not surprisingly, he played an important part in the development of the pharmaceutical industry, although others were also involved, particularly in the field of proprietary medicines. On the face of it, it seems only reasonable to believe that the apothecary gave rise to the dispensing chemist, but this has been denied by those much nearer in time than us to the meteoric rise of the chemist and druggist and dispensing chemist. John Mason Good, R. M. Kerrison, and Edward Harrison, crusading medical reformers and so perhaps not totally unprejudiced, have all written along these lines, but such limited research as has been done on the subject does not confirm their views, and the topic requires much more detailed work before any definite conclusion can be reached.

In contrast, much has been written about the apothecary's role in the rise of the medical general practitioner. There would seem to be little doubt that a section of the London Barbers' Company was, in the fourteenth and fifteenth centuries, practising not only surgery but also physic.[69] These barber-surgeons were given certain privileges, such as exemption from serving on juries, inquisitions, and assizes, and the Act of 1540 gave them immunity from bearing armour and service on watches. They probably, like their Continental counterparts, had exemption from the curfew as well. They were, in effect, the first general practitioners. Efforts were made to curtail their activities, to prevent their further incursion into the physicians' world. The London collegiate physicians were not so simplistic as to believe that their small numbers (around fifty for a population of 200,000 in 1600) could personally treat all those requiring medical attention; rather their battles were directed towards the establishment and maintenance of a medical hierarchy, and ensuring that their colleagues (whom they deemed to be auxiliaries), the barber-surgeons, surgeons, and apothecaries, did not by-pass them in their dealings with patients. Their greatest error

---

[69] Sharpe (editor), op. cit., note 44 above, Letter Book I, p. 135; J. F. South, *Memorials of the craft of surgery*, London, 1886, pp. 19, 22.

Margaret Pelling has stated that, ". . . the barbers, barbersurgeons and surgeons carried the main burden of general practice in the towns." ('Occupational diversity: barbersurgeons and the trades of Norwich, 1550–1640', *Bull. Hist. Med.*, 1982, **56**: 484–511, see p. 490.)

lay in not recognizing the necessity for, and the inevitable rise of, the general practitioner.

Why the development of the general practitioner in England should have become pre-eminently the responsibility of the apothecary and not the barber-surgeon (as was generally the case on the Continent) is not easy to decide. The rise of the apothecary to a position of power has been accredited to the rapid increase in the import of exotic drugs in the early seventeenth century, the popularity of the complex Galenic formulae, and above all, to the apothecaries' sound commercial practices and contacts. At any rate, it is to the apothecary as progenitor of the general practitioner that we turn first.

THE GENERAL PRACTITIONER

Zachary Cope wrote in 1961 that, "until recently", the general practitioner might be defined ". . . as one who practised medicine, surgery and midwifery, prescribed and in many instances dispensed medicines, and more than other members of the profession, had the continuous care of patients."[70] The introduction of the title "general practitioner" belongs to the nineteenth century, though this is not to say the species was not to be found at an earlier date. One of the earliest appearances of the title in print occurred in 1813, when Samuel Fothergill, in discussing the apothecary, wrote, "Those who practise pharmacy alone are few in number compared with those who exercise all branches of the profession. Every city, every town and almost every village in England and Wales presents one or more of these general practitioners. . . . "[71] He urged that they should not be known as apothecaries but that some other new designation be found. In this, he was supported by popular opinion. The term "general practitioner" by 1830 had come into such common usage that the Metropolitan Society of General Practitioners in Medicine and Surgery was instituted under the presidency of William Gaitskell, and the title "apothecary" is found only once in the first fifty pages of Robson's *London directory* (1854).

It is generally conceded that "it was chiefly from among the apothecaries that the general practitioner arose . . . " (Cope, p. 7), but his origins also lay with the surgeons, in particular those who had served in the army, navy, or the East India Company. Clark has noted that in the later eighteenth century the name "surgeon-apothecary" was coming into use, a term long favoured in Scotland (op. cit., footnote 7, p. 610). The amalgamation of these two branches was undoubtedly the trend of the times. In May 1761, John Aiken, lecturer at Warrington Academy, was endeavouring to settle his son in life, and wrote, ". . . we have therefore determined on physic, and as it grows pretty common to unite the two professions of apothecary and surgeon I could wish my son were placed where he has opportunities of learning both these branches,

---

[70] Sir Zachary Cope, 'The origin of the general practitioner', *Hist. Med.*, 1973, **5**: 3.

[71] Editorial, *Med. phys. J.*, 1813, **29**: 3–4. The term can, however, be found much earlier, though possibly with a slightly different connotation. In 1714, J. Bellers wrote of hospitals being useful ". . . to those physicians that are more general practitioners in Physick. . . ." He had noticed that there was a change in medical practice, for he wrote, "There are the same reasons for classing of Diseases, Medicine and Physicians, especially Chronicks and Acutes, as there was formerly to distinguish between physicians, chirurgeons and apothecaries . . . ." (*An essay towards the improvement of physic*, London, J. Sowle, 1914, pp. 10–11.)

though I would have the *principal attention* given to surgery and midwifery."[72] In fact, this union had been taking place for many a year but was only then being recognized.

There are many examples of the dual practice in earlier centuries. The Annals of the College of Physicians made reference to a man called Horseman, described as an apothecary and surgeon in 1723, and in 1658, Edward Randal, "chirurgo-pharmacopoeus" was accused of malpractice. Amongst the 294 licences issued in the diocese of London under the Act of 1511, from 1600 to 1725, there were three specifically for the combined practice of apothecary and surgeon, and nineteen for physicians or practitioners of physic and surgeons. Similar figures can be obtained from the subscription books of the same diocese; there were three such mixed practitioners from 1627 to 1644, and fifteen from 1663 to 1683.[73] The same picture can be seen in the diocese of Canterbury. Out of a total of 167 medical licences between 1568 and 1640, there were fifty-seven for physicians, 103 for surgeons, and seven for physicians and surgeons. Among those who signed the testimonials in 1605 were Nicholas Bennett, Theodore Beacon, Mr Spencer, and Robert Harvey, all of whom were "artis chirurgie professor et phisice professor".[74]

Pelling and Webster, in their survey of East Anglian medical practitioners, 1500–1640, concluded that "medical practice in London and the provinces was dominated by general practitioners, some licensed, most unlicensed. . . ." They cite as examples the John Cropps, father and son, who are mentioned in the Paston letters; Robert Hauust of Great Yarmouth with an ecclesiastical licence for medicine and surgery (1566); Philip Barrough, given a surgical licence by Cambridge in 1559 and one to practise medicine in 1572; as well as the three men who were awarded dual licences by the same university between 1540 and 1570.[75] Roberts has no doubt that there was widespread general practice in Tudor and Stuart England, and has shown that not only did apothecaries gain the right to practise medicine in Exeter in 1607, but that twelve licences for the practice of medicine and surgery were awarded in that diocese between 1568 and 1640.[76]

There is at least one example of mixed practice in the fifteenth century. In April 1462, William Hobbys was described as "the king's surgeon" in the household of Edward IV; by July 1470, he had been elevated to "principal surgeon of the body", but in 1475, he was referred to as "physicus et cirurgicus pro Corpore Regis".[77] In the time of Chaucer, Ussery has found six men who were both physicians and surgeons,

[72] Linnean Society, Pulteney letters, John Aiken senior to Richard Pulteney, 19 May 1761 (Aiken's italics).

[73] J. H. Bloom and R. R. James, *Medical practitioners in the diocese of London, licensed under the act 3 Henry VIII c. 21; an annotated list, 1529–1725*, Cambridge University Press, 1935. The three apothecaries and surgeons were Robert Hitchcox of Ware (1662), George de Folleville of Cheshunt, a French refugee (1693), and John Harris of Whitechapel, who was certified to have been admitted as a foreign brother to the Barber-Surgeons' Company.

Guildhall Library, MSS. 9539A/1, 9539/C, 9540/1, 9540/4. The licences for most but by no means all, of these subscribers to the ecclesiastical and political doctrines of the day are to be found in Bloom and James's list. There are also some differences, Ralph Warwick for example, on subscription was admitted to practise "artem chirurgie", but his licence was that for a physician.

[74] A. J. Willis (editor), *Canterbury licences (general) 1568–1646*, Chichester, Phillimore, 1972, pp. 22–29.

[75] Pelling and Webster, op. cit., note 29 above, pp. 235, 224, 195, 194.

[76] Roberts, op. cit., note 26 above, pp. 376, 369.

[77] A. R. Myers, *The household of Edward IV*, Manchester University Press, 1959, 2nd ed., p. 124 and n. 189, p. 29 and n. 191.

and quotes from Lanfranc, who wrote at the end of the fourteenth century, "... knowe wel this, that he is no good phisician that can no thing in cirurgie. And also the contrarie therof; and a man mai be no good cyrurgian but if he knowe phisik."[78]

Chief Justice Best said erroneously in 1828 that, "The distinction between the various departments of the medical art had been drawn with great precision", and two years later J. W. Willcock, "The law recognises only three orders of the medical profession: physicians, surgeons and apothecaries", so that Holloway was constrained to follow suit by writing, "Between the physician, who could claim to belong to a learned profession, the surgeon, who practised a craft, and the apothecary, who followed a trade, the gap was wide and impassable."[79] This was not true in the first decades of the nineteenth century, nor was it true in earlier years. The general practitioner has a long and respectable history.

The question arises, to what degree was the apothecary a component of the general practitioner's origins? We have on no less an authority than William Bulleyn that the Elizabethan apothecary was involved in surgical practice. His nineteenth rule, that the apothecary was to remember that he was only the physician's cook, has been quoted frequently, yet rules eleven and sixteen have caused less comment:

> 11. [The apothecary is] to have two places in his shop; one most cleane for the phisik, and a baser place for the chirurgie stuff.
> 16. That he may open wel a vein for to helpe pleurisy.[80]

The apothecaries' rules were published in Bulleyn's *Bulwarke of defence* in 1563, when he was practising in the ward of Cripplegate-without, London, so that he must have been aware of the privileges of the Barber-Surgeons' Company set out in the Act of 1540.

Roberts has shown that some apothecaries, for example John Swayton of Faversham in 1598 and Anthony Salter of Exeter in 1622, had licences for surgery, a definite step in the direction of general practice. William Dove, apothecary, was licensed at Exeter to practise both medicine and surgery in 1580, as were Thomas Flay and his apprentice James Collins, and John Pemberton of Liverpool to practise medicine. It was by no means unusual for apothecaries in the small towns of Berkshire, Herefordshire, Northamptonshire, Suffolk, and elsewhere to obtain medical licences, there being a particular upsurge in the 1630s in the time of Archbishop Laud. We have little direct evidence, but it is reasonable to assume that this medical practice embraced physic, at least simple surgery, and pharmacy.

Carter has noted that apothecaries were not required to subscribe to the Acts of Supremacy and Allegiance, nor were they mentioned as such in the Act of 1511.[81] Nevertheless, their letters testimonial for a licence to practise physic or surgery were

---

[78] H. E. Ussery, *Chaucer's physician*, New Orleans, Tulane University Press, 1971, p. 59.
[79] S. W. F. Holloway, 'Medical education in England, 1830–1858', *History*, 1964, **49**: 299–324, see p. 306.
[80] C. Townsend, 'Apothecaries, druggists and pharmacists, past, present and future', *Pharm. J.*, 1870, **11**: 615.
[81] E. H. Carter, *The Norwich subscription books*, London, Nelson, 1937, p. 134. There is a total absence of apothecaries in the visitation lists of the diocese of London, except for one cryptic note, "John Cook 'medicus' of Leigh. That he is an apothecary and served his apprenticeship and practised as such and not otherwise." See MS. 9537/24, f. 144v., note 83 below.

acceptable. On 25 April 1692, Joseph Freeman of Little Waltham, surgeon, was certified to be a competent practitioner by Benjamin Chamberlaine, licentiate in Chelmsford, apothecary, and William Swan, apothecary; likewise, Samuel Dale, botanist and apothecary at Braintree for thirty years, was one of the referees for John Clerke, of Castle Hedingham, apothecary and practitioner in physic, when he required a licence.[82]

The licences of vicars, schoolmasters, midwives, surgeons, and physicians were in theory checked by archidiaconal visitations. The visitations of the diocese of London for 1697, 1700, 1706, and 1715 are in good order, although only a section of the diocese was examined on each occasion. It is noticeable that within the City and nearby villages the vast majority of licences examined were those of surgeons. Ten or more miles distant, the situation was different; Staines in 1697 had two "medici", St Albans, one, and in 1706, Brentwood had one as well. Just what the authorities meant by "medicus" is not at all clear. Only two are specifically stated to have medical degrees, Benjamin Allen in Braintree, from Oxford, and Jonathan Bowes in Chelmsford, from Leiden. Ralph Grindale of Ware had a "Lambeth degree" (in other documents he is called "Dr in Physick"), and Rodon of Harwich a licence of London, otherwise no details are given.[83]

It is possible that many of those designated "medicus" were in fact apothecaries, and in two cases this can be proved. The previously mentioned John Clerke of Castle Hedingham was termed "medicus" at the visitation of 1715, on 1 September of the same year on making his subscription he was given leave to practice "artem medicinae", but on the 30th, as we have seen, he obtained his licence as an apothecary and practitioner in physic. Similarly, William Heckford of Thaxted showed his licence at the visitation, proving him to be "medicus et chir.", yet when he was taking apprentices in 1711 and 1724, he is described as an apothecary. A "medicus" could also be a surgeon, as witness John Holmsted of Colchester. In 1706, he made his subscription and obtained his licence as a surgeon, which he was termed in the visitation of that year, but in 1715, he was called "medicus". There was considerable inexactitude in the use of titles, and possibly it worried neither party that Robert Mayhew of Witham was a "medicus" in 1706 but had become a surgeon in 1715.[84]

It must not be thought that physic-practising apothecaries were not to be found in London before the Rose case or even before the Restoration. Roger Gwyn, apothecary to St Bartholomew's and St Thomas's hospitals, and the well-known and highly respected botanists, James Garrett, Hugh Morgan, and John Parkinson, were all prosecuted by the College of Physicians for illegal practice.

Roberts struck a note of caution in assuming that the apothecary-surgeon of the late seventeenth-century countryside developed entirely from the apothecary turned

[82] Bloom and James, op. cit., note 73 above, pp. 49, 43.

[83] Guildhall Library, Archidiaconal triennial visitations, MSS. 9537/24,9537/26. The accuracy of the scribes or perhaps their interpretation is doubted when it is noted that in Maldon in 1706 there was but one "medicus" and six surgeons, and yet only nine years later the situation is completely reversed with five "medici" and one surgeon – admittedly the two sets of names are different too.

[84] When Robert Ma[y]hew apprenticed his son in 1716 to Vesey Haslfoot (probably related to the Harwich surgeons, Robert and Thomas Haslfoot), citizen and goldsmith, his occupation was given as D[octor] of P[hysic].

medical practitioner. He felt that at least as much was owed to the surgeons, especially naval surgeons. The Inland Revenue apprenticeship records give some support to this view. They show a particularly high proportion of surgeons practising in and around the ports of Plymouth, Portsmouth, and Chatham. On a few occasions, the men are designated "surgeons etc.", which appears to be the scribes' shorthand for "surgeon and apothecary" or "surgeon, apothecary and man-midwife", for which the term "general practitioner" was ultimately substituted. The surgeons' oft-reiterated rejoinder that they had to give internal medicines without reference to a physician when at sea, was one which applied with equal force to surgeons living in distant lands that were being rapidly opened up to commercial development. The East India Company was well aware of the desirability of employing a man with all-round qualifications.

Edward Bulkeley, chirurgeon, was admitted to the London Barber-Surgeons' Company by redemption by order of Sir Henry Colt in September 1684.[85] He was appointed first surgeon to Fort St George (Madras) on 29 December 1692, when he was informed that he had been placed in charge of the hospital, that he was to take care of the patients, and ". . . look after all medicines and other things, that none be spoyled or wasted, or use for any other purpose. Keep an account of all material actions in a Book. Dr Brown is to be continued a Chyrurgion here as before . . . [but as there is] not roome for the continuance of Dr Hart, he is to be discharged". A communication from London informed Madras in April 1697 how this had come about. "When wee understood Mr Heathfield was dead and that you had entertained Mr Hart as a temporary surgeon in his stead, we resolved to supply you as soon as well as we could, and accordingly sent you Mr Buckley [*sic*] one who was every way very fitly qualified to serve us by his large experience of India as well as here, and as fit for prescribing Physick as manual operation."[86]

That Bulkeley was interested in the production of pharmaceuticals can be seen from his letters to James Petiver. He wrote on 12 February 1703, "I also desire you will send me ye waye of refining Camphir and sugar. We have brown sugars here very cheap, I want to refine them and make them into loafe. I want also the best and the easiest method of making Vinegar, we have often pricked and damaged wines but knowe not howe to make good vinegar of them, nor how to brighten that which is browne and fowle."[87]

Until the second half of the nineteenth century, complete reliance on the titles used can be completely misleading. As Roberts has written, "The point then is that it is necessary to get behind 'official' titles in administrative records to see how these men really did practise – for not only are the appellations misleading but also they were interchangeable. For example Thomas Edwards [originally an apothecary] having with difficulty become a physician in 1607, called himself 'surgeon' when his daughter applied for a marriage licence in 1623; John Newton was styled physician when he died in 1646 but he had been licensed by the Bishop in 1628 to practise surgery."

[85] Guildhall Library, admissions to Barber-Surgeons' Company, MS. 5265/2, f. 47.
[86] D. G. Crawford, *History of the Indian medical service, 1600–1913*, London, W. Thacker, 1914, p. 88, quoting from *Vestiges of old Madras*.
[87] British Library, Sloane MSS., MS. 3321, f. 110.

Clark, commenting on this Star Chamber case of 1604–07 examined by Roberts, wrote, "But it shows, and in conjunction with other known facts, that at and after this time the appellations of physician, apothecary, and for that matter surgeon and doctor, were not used either by provincial practitioners or in popular speech, or even in some official records, so as to demarcate different kinds of practice."[88]

Kett noted that, "After 1730 the words 'surgeon' and 'apothecary' were used interchangeably in the provinces. . . . Samuel Buxton was described as a 'worthy and sensible apothecary near the Wells' in 1769 and as 'Mr Buxton, surgeon' ten years later."[89] This view is borne out by a close examination of the Inland Revenue surgeons' and apothecaries' apprenticeships records. To men such as Anthony Harrison of Penrith (fl. 1743–83) and Henry Luximoore of Okehampton (fl. 1758–89) it seems to have been a matter of indifference as to whether they were termed surgeon, apothecary, or surgeon and apothecary; likewise with the Bryetts of Hatherleigh, Devonshire. In 1713, James Bryett was termed "Dr of Physick and surgeon", but in 1717 and 1721, just "surgeon". Thomas Bryett was "physician and surgeon" in 1730, and "surgeon etc." six years later.[90] This variation in title can be seen equally clearly if we follow the history of a medically orientated family such as the Oldershaws of Leicestershire.

The armigerous Oldershaw family lived in Kegworth in the fifteenth century, and the first apothecaries appeared on the scene towards the end of the seventeenth century. John and Fowler were the oldest and youngest sons of John Oldershaw JP and his wealthy wife Sarah (née Fowler), who lived at Old Parks, Loughborough.[91] John practised in his home town, and it is recorded that he had at least three apprentices; when he took William Fullwood in 1721, and John Robins of Salisbury, Wiltshire, he was entitled apothecary, but earlier, at the binding of Moses Foxcroft, apothecary and surgeon. John's second son, Francis, was sent to Emmanuel College, Cambridge, and there gained an MB in 1740, but he died the same year, aged only twenty-six. The next son, James, also entered medicine but by a different route, and in due course became established in Leicester. Nichols referred to him as a surgeon, but Emmanuel College, when his two sons were admitted (one to enter the church and the other, James, to acquire an MD in 1780), called him an apothecary. The apprenticeship records either agree with Nichols or give him the double title of apothecary and surgeon.[92] Whatever term was used, there is no doubt that by the time of his death in Rochester in 1782, he was a rich man.

Fowler Oldershaw left Loughborough for Market Bosworth and there set up in practice. His only recorded apprentice, when he was designated apothecary, was Theophilus, son of Henry Hastings of Thornton, Leicestershire, possibly a distant cousin of the earls of Huntingdon.[93] It is probable that Fowler trained two, if not

[88] Clark, op. cit., note 7 above, p. 608.

[89] J. F. Kett, 'Provincial medical practice in England, 1730–1815', *J. Hist. Med.*, 1964, **19**: 17.

[90] For further discussion see Burnby, op. cit., note 31 above, pp. 160–164.

[91] J. Nichols, *The history and antiquities of the county of Leicestershire*, London, [the author] 1798.

[92] Amongst James's apprentices was Francis Cheselden, a relative of the great William. Will of James Oldershaw of the City of Rochester, proved 2 May 1782, PRO, PCC, Prob. 11, 1091 f. 260.

[93] The second wife of Theophilus Hastings, the seventh earl, was Frances Leveson *Fowler*, and it is possible that there was a connexion. Their granddaughter, Elizabeth, Countess of Moira, wrote of a collateral branch of the Hastings, "His wife (a woman of very good family who was related to my

three, of his own sons. In his will of 1749 (he died aged fifty-seven), he made his oldest son John executor and bequeathed him "my shop and all druggs, materials and utensils belonging, also all my household goods and furniture in that house of which the said shop is part."[94a] John, who died some twelve years later, in his will of 1762, unlike his apothecary father, styled himself surgeon. He set up a trust for his only child, the trustees being his wife and his youngest brother, James, who was a surgeon in Tamworth.[94b]

James had already been elected a burgess of Tamworth in 1758, and was the founder of a successful medical practice. His first known apprentice was Walter Lyon in 1757, who was a partner ten years later when they became joint masters of James Henry Gresley; another of their apprentices was Edward Bage in 1770. On both occasions they were described as "surgeons etc.", a phrase which often included man-midwife, a branch of medicine it is known that they practised (see p. 107). James Oldershaw had retired by early 1788 when the firm was called Messrs. Lyon & Co., subsequently (1794) it became Messrs. Lyon and Bage, and then (1803) Bage & Woody, surgeons. Whatever title they used or was bestowed on them, the Oldershaws were, in fact, general practitioners, and had been for many a long year.

The administration of the English Poor Law must clearly also have had a considerable effect on the emergence and numbers of general practitioners. Leonard stated that, "A fairly effectual system of relieving the destitute by public authority had had in England a continuous existence since the seventeenth century. Attempts to follow such a system of poor relief in the sixteenth century were common to most of the countries of western Europe, but the continuous existence of any organization of the kind is peculiar to England."[95] Leonard believed that in large measure the survival of the English organization was due to the policy of the Privy Council in the reign of Charles I, which effectively interfered to enforce the administration by the justices of the peace of the Poor Law enacted in 1597 and practically re-enacted in 1601. The statutes of these two laws attempted to provide work for the unemployed, procure corn in years of bad harvests, regulate wages, and provide succour for the impotent poor, including the sick.

Provision was made for those who were struck down by illness or were victims of accidents. Leonard, writing at the very end of the nineteenth century, said, "In some places the help provided was even greater than that of today; a town physician was appointed especially to look after the poor." As early as 1574, the mayor and justices of Chester signed an indenture with Alexander Harrison, whereby the latter would "... cure, heale and help all such the poore deserved people ... within the citie living

---

grandmother and was her companion) . . . being a woman of independent spirit . . . wanted her husband to go into business. As he would not consent she undertook that task herself and thereby brought up and educated a large family. Her eldest son she put in the army; another in the law; and others in trades; all behaving respectably and succeeding in their different pursuits . . . ." See H. N. Bell, *The Huntingdon peerage case*, [privately published], 1820, p. 302.

[94] Lichfield Record Office, (a) will of Fowler Oldershaw of Market Bosworth, apothecary, proved 10 February 1750; (b) will of John Oldershaw of Market Bosworth, surgeon, proved 22 March 1763. His son John was admitted to St Mary Hall, Oxford, in June 1776; he became BCL in 1783, DCL in 1819, and vicar of Tarvin, Cheshire.

[95] E. M. Leonard, *The early history of English poor relief*, Cambridge University Press, 1900, preface, p. vii.

upon the almes of the citie of all their ulcers, wounds, sickness, and deseases etc." A surgeon in Newcastle upon Tyne received forty shillings in 1592 as his accustomed fee for helping ". . . to cure the maimed poor folk"; in later years he came to be known as the town physician, and by 1632, a Mr Henderson was receiving £20 as a half-yearly stipend. Barnstaple was equally provident, in November 1629 engaging a Dr Symes at £20 a year.[96]

This assistance to the sick poor was one of the sections of the Elizabethan Poor Law that survived into the Restoration and beyond;[97] vestry minutes or the accounts of the overseers of the poor afford many examples. Whittet and Newbold have shown that Peter Dent, William Frisby, Edmund Halfhyde, Artemas Hinds, and Charles Gilman, all apothecaries of Cambridge, were paid by the overseers in the parishes of St Peter's, St Edward's, and Great St Mary's between 1685 and 1707.[98] Although Newcastle talked of its "townes physitian", Barnstaple referred to a "learned physician" being employed, and Cavendish, Suffolk, commissioned Richard Hawes in 1758 as their "physician and surgeon", most towns made use of apothecaries or surgeons as their medical practitioners. The towns of Eaton Socon and Enfield, Middlesex, may be taken as typical examples.

The first medical practitioners noted in the accounts of Eaton Socon and the nearby village of Roxton were a Dr Trott and a Dr Williams, both of St Neots, Huntingdonshire.[99] Although both men were accorded the honorary title of "doctor", neither had a degree. The former was John Trott, son of Edward, clerk, who had been bound in 1688 to Joseph Pawlett, citizen and apothecary of London.[100] From 1702 to 1721, he was employed at different times by the authorities of Roxton and Eaton Socon. Trott had at least four apprentices, one of whom, Samuel Archdeacon, was to be employed by the parish from 1758 onwards. Dr Williams was George Williams, described in the apprenticeship records as either a "surgeon" or "surgeon etc.". His bills could be sizeable. In 1724, he received £11 10s. 6d. for setting and "cureing" William Bass's leg, and when Widow Gazeley's boy required the same treatment, the bill was settled in two halves, one in 1707 and the other two years later.

Others, such as Drs Jesham, Appleby, King, and Rolt, came from St Neots as occasion demanded, and so did James Crow, possibly a barber-surgeon, as he dealt primarily in phlebotomies and salves. Specialist treatment was also sought from Mr Fisher, the bonesetter. The "wise women" were paid small sums for dealing with sore hands, burns, and scald heads.

At first, the medical bills were paid as and when they occurred, but by the second quarter of the eighteenth century, medical contracts began to be made, possibly as a result of the high expenses that had been incurred. A vestry resolution of 19 January 1730 stated that the parish of Eaton Socon had agreed to pay £5 ". . . from this time . . . to Easter 1731 [to] Mr John Sharpe, an apothecary [who] shall find all

[96] Ibid., p. 202, quoting Welford's *Newcastle and Gateshead*, p. 132, and 'Wyot's diary', *North Devon Herald*, 21 April 1881.

[97] E. G. Thomas, 'The old poor law and medicine', *Med. Hist.*, 1980, **24**: 1–19. Vivian Nutton, review of Webster (editor), op. cit., note 29 above, in ibid., 471–473.

[98] Whittet and Newbold, op. cit., note 52 above, pp. 115–118.

[99] F. G. Emmison, 'The relief of the poor at Eaton Socon, 1706–1834', *Beds. Hist. Rec. Soc.*, 1933, **15**: 1–99, see pp. 78–79.

[100] Guildhall Library, Apothecaries' Society court minutes, MS. 8200/2, f. 260.

manner of surgery and physick for all the poor of our said parish . . .". Dr Sharpe's bills for 1729 had amounted to £28, so the parish was being distinctly hopeful, not to say parsimonious, to contain the costs to this low sum. Indeed, it was obviously impossible, as when the contract ran out, the next was made with a "Mr Willis Atkins" [Adkins] for six guineas a year. He had been frequently called in by the overseers from 1718 onwards.

These men practised not only as apothecaries and surgeons, but also as man-midwives. From 1709 to 1719, Eaton Socon made nineteen disbursements for lyings-in. Usually, only the midwife was paid her half-crown fee, but sometimes the doctor was also present, as for example, "To Dr Williams for doeing his office in laying Musgrave's wife. £3 4s. 6d.". Successors to Willis Adkins were Jonathan and William Gorum (or Goreham), thought to be uncle and nephew), Samuel Archdeacon and his son, Robert Vickery, and William Halliley, all of whom are known to have been either surgeons or surgeons and apothecaries.[101]

The vestry minutes and parochial charity records for the small but wealthy market town of Enfield, Middlesex, are not extant before the last quarter of the seventeenth century, consequently the first reference to parish medical aid dates from 1682.[102] On 24 September of that year, a Mr Huddleston received £2 10s. for "cureing a poor man called Jeremiah Gillam". John Huddleston was the son of Robert, a fellmonger, a man of some means as his will shows.[103] John was apprenticed to Henry Cliff of the London Barber-Surgeons' Company in 1665, and probably spent most of his professional life there; this was the sole occasion he was called in by the parish, and it may well have been at the behest of his brother, Robert junior, who was one of Enfield's schoolmasters.[104]

The next man to appear was Robert Murrell in 1684, who received £4, "for curing the wife of John Mountegue, a husbandman, living in Green Street whose leg was dangerously broken". In subsequent years, Murrell appeared frequently for ever larger sums of money; the charity minutes for 5 August 1709 have the entry "Paid Mr Murrell for the cure of a mans head and arm wounded by the Mill, for the cure of Grace Saxbeys leg, for the cure of Wid. Ingles arm and for the cure of John Smedleys leg. £15". Two years later, he was paid £11 9s., and a note was added, "More due to him £26 11s.".[105] Murrell's work seems to have been mainly, if not entirely, concerned with surgery. He probably trained his son William in the same art with the idea of him succeeding to the practice, as in the visitation of 1715 it is William Murrell who is named surgeon for Enfield and not Robert as in 1697.[106] When he made his will in

[101] Emmison, op. cit., note 99 above.

[102] Thomas Greenhill, apothecary, was in Enfield between the years 1660 and 1677, and may have tended the parish poor. John Stephens, chyrurgeon, was in the town from 1678 onwards, but neither he nor his son Benjamin, apothecary, are known to have been employed by the parish.

[103] Guildhall Library, Commissary Court wills, MS. 9171/35, f. 289, 13 July 1675.

[104] Ibid., Barber-Surgeons' Company bindings, MS. 5266/1, f. 109r; Robert Huddlestone, in his will dated April 1713, referred to him as ". . . my brother John citizen and chirurgeon of London now living at Enfield".

[105] Vestry minutes and Enfield parochial charities' accounts held in the vestry of St Andrew's Church, Enfield.

[106] Robert Murrell married three times. William, born January 1683, was the son of his first wife, Mary. Richard, the son of his third marriage, was apprenticed in 1736, after his father's death, to Daniel Harper, surgeon of St Mary's, Whitechapel.

October 1728, Robert termed himself surgeon, but he had other sources of income. The survey of the manor of Enfield, 1686, shows that he held nearly forty acres of demesne land, rented from the feoffees a tenement known as the Greyhound, part of John David's gift, and held a freehold messuage in Bridge Street. He seems to have disposed of most of this property before his death, but, nevertheless, held two messuages and a brewhouse in Silver Street.[107]

The Enfield charities paid out sums of money to lay persons such as Thomas Maskall in 1695 (£5), Robert Smithson in 1700 (£5), Mr John Game 50s. in 1685 and a further 50s. was promised if his cure was successful, Margaret Crisp for treating four children troubled with scald heads (£2), the Widow Mountegue for a cure done to John Welch (£2 10s), and there were, of course, the midwifery cases. Sarah Fish receiving £1 3s. 6d. in 1701. A Thomas Jones was in receipt of three sums of money. It is possible that he was a bonesetter and manipulator who specialized in ruptures, although when his two sons were apprenticed, he was described as a gentleman.[108]

Another man who was much employed was Thomas Wilford, and there is no doubt that he was an apothecary. Thomas was baptised at St Andrew's, the parish church of Enfield, on 13 October 1651, the son of Edward and Susan Wilford, members of an influential, well-to-do, and educated local family. When Thomas was sixteen, his father exchanged indentures with William Phillips, citizen and apothecary of London, for his son to have an eight-year apprenticeship, starting on Lady Day 1669.[109] It is probable that Wilford first of all practised in London, but certainly from 1704 onwards he treated the poor of Enfield. It is apparent from the charity minutes that he was practising as both physician and surgeon. In November 1705, he received £2 6s. "for physick given to several poor", and there is still extant a bill of his dated 1709, "For performing a cure on Goody Roberts leg, which had been very bad for above a year by Poultesses, Fomentations, Oyntments, Plasters and several bottles of dyett drink, for all which we deserve no less than forty shillings. Thomas Wilford." Goody's leg was still giving trouble in 1714, and Thomas was still hopefully "cureing" it.

Thomas Wilford died in 1719, the year in which the workhouse came into being. Who immediately followed him and Robert Murrell in their attendance on the poor is not known, as the records are defective, but from 1744 a Joseph Wilson was receiving £21 a year ". . . for his salary as Surgeon and Apothecary to the Parish."[110] He was also given one or two guineas for "attending a woman in labour" or "laying a woman". Other records show that Wilson was as comfortably placed in life as Robert

---

[107] PRO, Duchy of Lancaster records, survey of the manor of Enfield, 1686, MS. DL 43/7/9; Guildhall Library, Commissary Court wills, MS. 9168/36, 6 March 1733.

[108] In 1713 and 1714, Thomas Jones apprenticed Thomas (baptized 1696) and John (baptized 1699) to two men whom the clerk of the Inland Revenue office termed citizens and barber-surgeons. The Company records, however, are more explicit. Thomas's master, John Kirkham, is called a surgeon but John's, Richard Frisby, a "consarcinator" (?consigner). Later, it is recorded that John Jones, apprentice of Richard Frisby, barber, was turned over to Samuel Seddon, packer. To confuse matters further, Richard Frisby proves to have been bound in 1692 to a William Curtis, packer, and then turned over to Jacob Wilson, "libert. cloath-worker". An example of the way in which official documents, whilst not totally incorrect, may be misleading.

[109] Guildhall Library, Apothecaries' Society court minutes, MS. 8200/2, f. 123v; made free 4 September 1677, f. 224r.

[110] His licence to practise, obtained 26 November 1724, describes him as "Joseph Wilson of Enfield. surgeon". See Bloom and James, op. cit., note 73 above, p. 35.

Murrell or Thomas Wilford. He was in possession of three dwellings in Enfield and rented a fourth, the mansion house of Ridlingtons in which he lived. In addition, he had several large parcels of land, a brewhouse, and, for a short period, the Two Brewers public house at Ponders End.[111] His daughter Catherine, in 1761, married a surgeon, John Cameron, who succeeded to his father-in-law's practice.[112]

It is probable that Cameron continued to attend the poor for some years, but he must have relinquished the service by 1772, as the vestry minutes record that in November 1774, Thomas Prichard was given £21 as a year's salary "…for attending the poor as Doctor due at Mich. 1773." Prichard, a surgeon, had been in Enfield since at least 1755, when he figured in the rates book, and the following year received two guineas from the parish for delivering Hall's wife. In 1775, he was joined by John Sherwen, and their combined salary was increased to £31 10s. Sherwen, like Prichard and Wilson, was an "incomer", and received his initial training from Anthony Harrison, apothecary of Penrith.[113]

In any study of the development of the general practitioner, it is instructive to investigate the history of a modern firm of doctors from its recent past to its origins, so tracing its growth and studying the men who participated in it.

The medical practice in Church Street, Edmonton, endured for two hundred years, and even now is to be found "just round the corner". The first record of its existence can be dated to May 1733, when Robert Killingly presented a bill to the committee of the new workhouse. Unhappily for him, they voted against payment, probably because only a fortnight earlier they had appointed Dr Swift "to be our Physician & Apothecary" at £12 a year. Nine years later, however, it was agreed that "Mr Killingly be the Parish Apothecary" at the same salary, an offer which he accepted.[114] Robert had been apprenticed to William Beckington, citizen and apothecary of London in 1722, but never applied for the freedom of the Society, possibly because he intended to practise just on the seven-mile boundary outside the City.[115]

Killingly died in 1755, and he was followed in his practice by John Hammond, who married his daughter Frances two years later. It is not known where Hammond was

[111] London Borough of Enfield local history library, courts baron of manor of Worcesters, 1750 and 1758; Trinity College Library, Cambridge, Tithe map of 1754; Greater London Record Office, court baron of manor of Durants, 1753. In 1749, the Window Tax assessments for the first and second quarters show he owed tax on sixty-six windows.

[112] London Borough of Enfield local history library. The Eliab Breton sale of 1771, "An apothecary's shop, wash house, stable etc. let to Mr Cameron on lease of which 32 years unexpired."

[113] PRO, Inland Revenue apprenticeship records, I.R./1/56, f. 15. Sherwen received further short periods of training at Edinburgh and St Thomas's Hospital, London. He passed as a surgeon to an Indiaman on 1 June 1769, and made at least one voyage to the Far East. He became an MD (Aberdeen) in 1798 and an extra-licentiate of the London College of Physicians in 1802. He was a Shakespearian scholar, was involved in the Rowley/Chatterton controversy, and was himself a poet of no mean attainment. For further details of his career, see J. Burnby, *John Sherwen and drug cultivation in Enfield*, Edmonton Hundred Historical Society, Occasional Paper No. 23, 1973.

[114] London Borough of Enfield local history library. Edmonton workhouse committee minutes for May 1733, unpaginated; Edmonton vestry minutes for April 1742.

[115] Guildhall Library, Apothecaries' Society court minutes, MS. 8200/5, f. 56v. The will of Robert Killingly shows that he possessed several copyhold tenements in Church Street, Edmonton. The Killinglys seem to have been well placed in life; his aunt, Frances Hankin of Hornsey, bequeathed his family silverware in 1742, and the will of his son, Robert, shows that he traded with Antigua and probably lived there for a period.

trained, but the chances are high that his master was Killingly. Hammond was a successful man, a close friend of Sir James Winter Lake, governor of the Hudson Bay Company, and Pierce Galliard of Bury Hall; he appointed Lake trustee for his will of 1790, in which he described himself as an apothecary and surgeon. He bequeathed his three sons, William, Thomas, and John, £1,200 to be equally divided, and earnestly desired that they should ". . . continue together and to aid and assist each other to the utmost of their respective powers in carrying on their business of Surgeons and Apothecarys."[116] Shortly after his death, the Edmonton vestry passed the motion ". . . respecting a vacancy of an apothecary in room of the late Mr John Hammond, it was unanimously resolved that Mr William Hammond and Mr Thomas Hammond, be continued as apothecaries of the Parish on the same terms . . . viz. £50 a year but to find every kind of Medicine and to be subject to be discharged on non-attendance in their duty to the poor."

William and Thomas had been trained by their father before they went to Guy's Hospital as dressers to William Lucas in 1781 and 1786. The details for John are missing, but it is known that he attended Guy's Hospital (or possibly St Thomas's Hospital) in 1791. All three sons passed the diploma of the London Company of Surgeons.[117] Despite their father's stated wishes, the three young men soon went their separate ways. John was already in Enfield by 1795, and there married the daughter of a neighbour, William Complin, a well-established surgeon and apothecary who earlier had been in practice in Goodmansfields near the Royal Mint.[118] William Hammond stayed within the parish of Edmonton but removed himself to its most rural point on the edge of Enfield Chase, now known as Southgate. Like his father, he trained his own son, another William, and then sent him to be a dresser to Astley Cooper.[119] From the will of the older William, proved in 1837, we learn not only that father and son had drawn up articles of co-partnership in a "business as a surgeon and apothecary", but that they also had a shop well stocked with drugs.

The Church Street practice continued to be run by Thomas Hammond, the middle brother, whose greatest claim to fame is that he was the apprentice-master of John Keats. Of his three sons, two, Henry Samuel and Edward Bowles, chose the same career as their father and uncles. The younger boy, a contemporary and probably fellow-apprentice of Keats, gained his MRCS at the second attempt in 1819. He then practised in one of his father's branch surgeries in nearby Fore Street until his early death.[120] Henry Samuel was not his father's apprentice but

[116] PRO, PCC, Prob. 11 1192, f. 240.

[117] Archive office, Guy's Hospital Medical School, registers of entry of physicians' and surgeons' dressers, 1778–1813, Guy's and St. Thomas's Hospitals pupils and dressers, 1755–1823; Royal College of Surgeons' Library, Examination book of the Company of Surgeons, William Hammond, June 1783, Thomas Hammond, May 1787, John Hammond, March 1795.

[118] William Complin returned to London and died at Spital Square in 1808. He bequeathed to his son-in-law, Nicholas Birch, surgeon, all his books of physic and surgery, and to his son, Edward, druggist, all ". . . my books of herbals and dispensary".

[119] It was probably through her brother that Ann Elisha Hammond met and married in 1813 Joseph Henry Green, the celebrated demonstrator at Guy's Hospital who made the famous introduction between the two poets, Keats and Coleridge.

[120] From 1826, Edward Bowles Hammond was in partnership with Henry Biddle, surgeon, who was five years his junior. The firm was still known as Hammond and Biddle in 1837, nine years after Edward's death; it finally became Henry Biddle and Son.

was indentured with the well-known surgeon Thomas Blizard at a premium of 200 guineas.[121] He became MRCS in 1814 (and FRCS in 1858), and on his father's death three years later took over the Church Street practice. In 1842, exactly a hundred years after Robert Killingly's appointment as parish apothecary, Henry Samuel became medical officer to the Edmonton Poor Law Union at £110 a year.

Henry had a large family but only the youngest son, Samuel, decided on medicine as a career. Samuel took the double qualification of MRCS and LSA in 1858, and was the first of the family to become a licentiate of a Royal College of Physicians (Edinburgh) in 1860. The following year, he left Edmonton, not to return.[122] This must have been a blow to his father, who in 1862, when he was seventy, took into partnership a young surgeon with the resounding name of Charles James Massey Morris. Four years later, Henry Samuel retired and Morris succeeded to the practice, where he was to remain for another thirty years. The Church Street firm of doctors did not move until 1931, when the old house was demolished.

The history of a present-day firm of general practitioners having thus been followed, it is equally worthwhile to scrutinize the history of a strongly medically-orientated family. The changes of title and of education in each generation reveal the manner in which the practitioner of today has grown out of the surgeon or apothecary of the early eighteenth century.

The central figure at the beginning of this story was John Snashall, son and grandson of maltsters in Lewes, Sussex, who was apprenticed to Richard Russell, surgeon of the same town, in 1713.[123] In 1730, Snashall rebuilt 203 High Street, and practised there for the next thirty-six years. He married for the second time, Mary Ridge, widow of Thomas Ridge of Southover, but there were no children. An apprentice of his, Joseph Ridge (1734–1816), son of a woollen-draper and a distant relative of Mary, inherited the practice in the High Street.[124] To cement matters further, Joseph married Snashall's niece. John Snashall is known to have had at least six apprentices when he was termed either surgeon or apothecary, to which titles Joseph Ridge added man-midwife.

At an unknown date, Ridge took in a partner, an apothecary known as Dr John Chambers, who became the apprentice-master of Ridge's nephew Thomas (1760–1822) in 1775. This Thomas was the first of the Ridges who left Lewes to gain experience in a hospital, but was by no means the last. He began attending courses at Guy's Hospital in 1781, to be followed in 1798 by Samuel, the son of Joseph Ridge who had given him his preliminary training. Thomas then went to Great Yarmouth, where he practised until his death in 1822.

This history of the Ridge medical connexions now takes a slight shift to another

---

[121] It is possible that Thomas Hammond and Thomas Blizard were personal friends, as Hammond's youngest daughter was baptized Harriet Blizard in August 1808.

[122] For further details of the Hammond family see, J. Burnby, *The Hammonds of Edmonton*, Edmonton Hundred Historical Society, Occasional Paper No. 26, 1973.

[123] There were a number of medical Russells in Lewes; this Richard is probably the one nicknamed "Sea Water Russell", son of Nathaniel, an apothecary, and who after an advantageous marriage obtained an MD at Leiden in 1724. See T. D. Whittet, 'Apothecaries and the development of sea bathing', *Pharm. Hist.*, 1981, **11**: no. 3, 7–8.

[124] For much of this material I am indebted to Dr Jessie Ridge of Seaford, Sussex.

PEDIGREE OF SNASHALL & RIDGE FAMILIES*

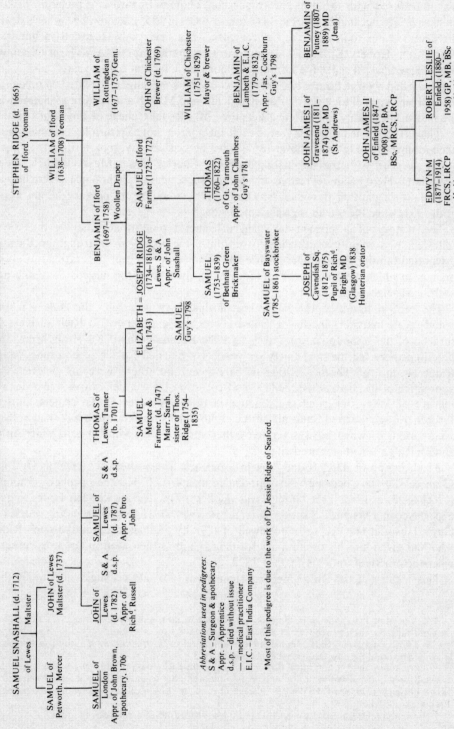

Abbreviations used in pedigrees:
S & A – Surgeon & apothecary
Appr. – Apprentice
d.s.p. – died without issue
—– medical practitioner
E.I.C. – East India Company

*Most of this pedigree is due to the work of Dr Jessie Ridge of Seaford.

38

branch.[125] Benjamin (1779–1832), son of William Ridge, brewer and brandy merchant, mayor of Chichester and second cousin to the previously mentioned Thomas, was apprenticed in 1795 to James Cockburne, "surgeon etc." of the same city for six years. Benjamin did not complete his apprenticeship, for he had joined Samuel Ridge at Guy's Hospital by 1798. Two years later, he joined the East India Company as a ship's surgeon. He did not lead the roaming life for long, because he was settled in Lambeth in 1802.

Of Benjamin's four sons, the two younger decided not only to enter medicine but that formal qualifications were then the order of the day. The elder, Benjamin II (1807–89), became first an LSA, then an MD (Jena, 1839), and an FRCS (1854). He was the author of many medical papers. The younger brother, John James (1811–74), after experience with his father, went to Guy's Hospital as family tradition demanded, finally gaining the double qualification MRCS, LSA, and an MD (St Andrews 1852). J.J., as he was called, practised as a general practitioner in Gravesend, Kent, where he became a justice of the peace and mayor. He was of an inventive turn of mind and took out a number of patents, the most successful being "Dr Ridge's patent food". The Post Office Directory lists him as being both a surgeon and a chemist and druggist in 1862, a description that was far from inaccurate, because he was the first chairman of the General Apothecaries' Company, which existed from 1856 to 1959.[126] A broadsheet informed the public that the company's avowed intention was to supply ". . . unadulterated Drugs and Chemicals, Invalid Foods, Condiments, Sanatory [*sic*] and Domestic Articles; to prepare Physician and other Prescriptions, Photographic Chemicals etc." The directors claimed they had fitted up extensive laboratories and drug mills and employed "Scientific Chemists" for the testing and analysis of all goods sold. All of this is a reminder of general practitioners' apothecarial forebears.

It is unnecessary to follow this medically-centred family further, except to say that J.J.'s only son J.J.II (BA, BSc, MRCS, LRCP, MD(Lond.)), a general practitioner in Enfield and co-founder of the Cottage Hospital, was the father of two doctors (MB BCh(Edin.), and FRCS, LRCP), grandfather of two more (both MB BS), and great-grandfather of another (MB BS, MRCGP), general practitioners in Enfield to this day. From this can be seen the steps taken in one family from eighteenth-century apothecary to member of the Royal College of General Practitioners.

There is no doubt that the apothecary was an essential factor in the genesis of the general practitioner, but it is equally obvious that the title "apothecary" was not an exact one. Throughout the eighteenth century and even earlier, the terms "surgeon" and "apothecary" could scarcely be differentiated in the provinces. John Trott and Thomas Wilford were both apprenticed to London apothecaries; neither, as far as is known, had training with a surgeon, and yet both worked as the mixed practitioners of the day in Eaton Socon and Enfield. Possibly, the London apothecary practised far more surgery than is generally supposed, a view that gains greater credence when the education of Samuel Snashall, cousin of the previously mentioned John, is considered. On 4 June 1706, Samuel, the son of a mercer of Petworth, Sussex, was bound for eight years to John Brown, a member of the London Society of Apothecaries. Surprisingly,

---

[125] See Snashall and Ridge pedigree.
[126] T. D. Whittet, 'The Liverpool Apothecaries' Company', *Chem. Drugg.*, 1965, **184**: 40–41.

he did not seek the freedom of that Company but rather that of the Barber-Surgeons, "1 February 1715, Samuel Snashall, chirurgeon, apprentice of John Browne, foreign brother, admitted by redemption. Paid £3 4s. 6d."[127] When cases such as this are explored, it becomes increasingly apparent that many of the barriers erected by historians between the London guilds are artificial and fragile.

It is also true to say that the implementation of the Poor Laws was instrumental in the emergence of the general practitioner. The apothecary, skilled in physic and pharmacy, and with some surgical expertise, practised, as occasion demanded, the neglected and despised expertise of midwifery. Neither was this just a second-rate service fit only for the lower orders. Dr Joan Lane, working on Warwickshire material for the years 1750–1834, has found that apprenticeship as a means of training was held in very high esteem, and that the parish poor and the gentry were treated by the same medical practitioners.[128]

THE EXPERIMENTAL AND MANUFACTURING CHEMIST

Chemistry as a science in its own right with its own individual approach to problems, its own technology and concepts, is a late product of the Scientific Revolution. The work of Dalton, Lavoisier, Cavendish, Priestley, and Black established chemistry as a clearly defined branch of science; any attempt to classify earlier sources that led to both chemical theory and practice immediately becomes complex. Discoveries in mineralogy or physics, in metallurgy or biology, could have chemical significance; even more obviously related were developments in industrial technology and medicine. A. R. Hall has written that, "By the end of the seventeenth century the best accounts of experimental chemistry were those written with medical applications in mind", adding that such progress was due to ". . . physicians and apothecaries, among them Boerhaave, Cullen, Scheele and Black."[129] The teaching of chemistry began in the universities around 1700 but only as an adjunct to medicine, and even at the end of the century, when Black was lecturing at Edinburgh the bulk of his listeners were medical students.

The study of chemistry by medical practitioners gained its greatest impetus from the works of Paracelsus and his followers; the English Paracelsian, Noah Biggs, in 1651, went so far as to call for a "Reformation of the Universities and the whole Landscap of Physick", which would thus effect the discovery of the "Terra incognita of Chymistrie".[130] The replacement of the humoral theory by the three principles, sulphur, salt, and mercury, was no advance in medical theory, nor was the esoteric Paracelsian and Helmontian philosophy in any degree helpful to medical practice, but these physicians had the effect of promoting chemically-prepared medicines and the analysis of mineral waters. As Franklin has written, "The physicians were at liberty to spin their webs of intuitive chemical thought, but for the apothecaries and druggists whose livelihood depended on their ability to market drugs, the improvement of

[127] Guildhall Library, Apothecaries' Society court minutes, MS. 8200/4, f. 247; Freedoms of the Barber-Surgeons' Company, MS. 5265/4, f. 61.
[128] Dr Joan Lane, Centre for the Study of Social History, University of Warwick. Personal communication.
[129] A. R. Hall, *The scientific revolution, 1500–1800*, London, Longmans, 1962, p. 320.
[130] A. G. Debus, 'Paracelsian medicine: Noah Biggs and the problem of medical reform', in Debus (editor), op. cit., note 6 above, p. 36.

chemical procedures had become a practical necessity".[131]

Two immensely popular works were produced in the early years of the seventeenth century to cater for this demand, Oswald Croll's *Basilica chymica* and Jean Beguin's *Tyrocinium chymicum*. Later in the century, these books were followed by those of Nicasius Le Febvre, Christopher Glaser, Moise Charas, and Nicolas Lemery.[132] By 1685, advertisements such as that of Thomas Hammond's could be seen, ". . . sundry select and experimental Medicines such whose Beneficence is well known to the most eminent Physicians, faithfully prepared and sold by Thomas Hammond, at his house, the sign of the Blew Balls in Ave-Mary Lane, leading from Lud Gate Street to Pater Noster Alley, who has been practically conversant as well as Studient in Chymical Pharmacy . . . above ten years past". His list of preparations included: (i) "The Queen of Hungary's Water"; (ii) "The English Orvietan or the curious purging antidote"; (iii) "The Elixir proprietatis, impregnated with volatile salt of Hartshorn"; (iv) "The Tincture of the Salt of Tartar (of a Rubicund colour)"; (v) "The ponderous Acid Oyle of Vitriol made Volatil and sweet"; (vi) "Dullidge Water evaporated so as a Pint will Purge as much as three Quarts crude from the Well."[133] Thomas Hammond has not been found to be a member of the Society of Apothecaries; nor was his contemporary, George Wilson (1631–1711), a chemist of greater note. Wilson received his freedom of the Company of Haberdashers by order of the Court of Aldermen, and in his will referred to himself as "citizen and haberdasher". Nothing is known of his origins, but he was certainly established at the sign of the Hermes Trismegistus, Watling Street in the parish of St Mary Aldermary, by the time of the Great Plague, during which he was kept exceedingly busy. About 1688, he moved to Well Yard, near St Bartholomew's Hospital, and there he wrote his *Compleat course of chymistry* printed in 1691. It formed the basis of many public lectures from then until well into the eighteenth century.[134] It was an eminently practical book and contained chapters on how to "lute limbeckes", "terms used in chymistry", how "to fortifie cracked glass", how to "defend a glass in a naked flame" by means of pipe clay or jackets of sand, besides sections on Dr Starkey's pill, "Matthew's his pill", extract of Peruvian bark, amber, extract of opium, and sugar.[135]

The book seems to have been intended to be used in conjunction with his most successful courses in chemistry. They were advertised in John Houghton's weekly paper, *A collection for the improvement of husbandry and trade,* in 1694, which

[131] A. W. Franklin, 'Clinical medicine', in ibid., p. 125. See also, C. Webster, *The great instauration. Science, medicine and reform, 1626–1660*, London, Duckworth, 1975; N. G. Coley, ' "Cures without care". "Chymical physicians" and mineral waters in seventeenth-century English medicine', *Med. Hist.*, 1979, **23**: 191–214.

[132] Nicasius Le Febvre, *A compendious body of chymistry*, London, 1662, "Apothecary in ordinary and Chymical distiller to the King of France and at present to his Majesty of Great Britain". Christoper Glaser, *The compleat chymist, a new treatise of chymistry*, London 1677; Glaser was a Swiss who held the chair of chemistry at the Jardin des Plantes. Moise Charas, *Pharmacopée royale galénique et chymique*, Paris, 1676 (London 1678); a master apothecary, who was successor to Glaser. Nicolas Lemery, *Cours de Chymie*, Paris, 1675; a French apothecary.

[133] British Library, advertisement of Thomas Hammond, 546.d.44(11).

[134] F. W. Gibbs, 'George Wilson, (1631–1711)', *Endeavour*, 1953, **12**: 183.

[135] George Starkey was one of the "chymical physicians" who did not survive the Great Plague; before his death, he imparted the formula for his pill, the compound soap pill, which found its way into the London Pharmacopoeia of 1746. He sold an earlier variant to Matthews.

informs us that the lectures and demonstrations were held in Wilson's house and that a full course cost three guineas. Others who followed his example and methods were Edward Bright, a chemist with a laboratory in Whitefriars near Fleet Street, and William Johnson at the sign of Van Helmont's Head in Fetter Lane. Johnson had been employed by Robert Boyle and had a knowledge of both physics and chemistry.

The Honourable Robert Boyle (1627–91) stands squarely at the watershed of chemical thought and theory. Although Boyle is often dubbed "the father of chemistry", John Freind in his chemical lectures in 1704 at Oxford was rather more correct when he commented that ". . . he had not so much laid down a new Foundation of Chymistry, as he had thrown down the old".[136] Boyle went to Oxford in 1655, and there lodged with John Crosse, an apothecary, thereby following the example of William Petty (1623–87), who had lived at the house of another apothecary, Arthur Tillyard.[137] Boyle soon employed Robert Hooke to be his chemical operator, and in January 1660 brought over the German chemist, Peter Stähl, to act as demonstrator. Stähl began to teach chemistry to any that were interested, and many took advantage of the opportunity, including the mathematicians Christopher Wren and John Wallis, and the physicians Ralph Bathurst, Thomas Millington, and Richard Lower. What is not known is whether the apothecaries, besides providing facilities, participated further in these chemical experiments. It is possible that Stephen Toone did so, because he and three Oxford surgeons, Francis Smith, William Day, and John Gill, were all close friends of John Ward when he was studying medicine and the allied disciplines of chemistry, botany, and physiology in the years between 1650 and 1668.[138]

Pilkington has pointed out that Boyle could with justice be regarded as a director of an extensive private institution.[139] Amongst those who worked for and with him were the previously mentioned Robert Hooke and Peter Stähl, Denis Papin, Hugh Greg, Frederick Slare, and another German, Ambrose Godfrey Hanckwitz. Boyle moved to London in 1668, the capital having become the centre of scientific thought, and there set up new laboratories in Maiden Lane. It is often said that Hanckwitz helped Boyle in the erection of the building, but as all the evidence of Hanckwitz's birth points to it being in 1660, this is clearly impossible. He was born at Nienburg, and it is not known when he came to this country or how Boyle came to know him, but it is very likely to have been before 1683, the probable date of the birth of his eldest son, Boyle Godfrey Hanckwitz. Again, what training Ambrose (I) had in chemistry is far from clear, although from his own testimony he served a Mr Steiger, chymist, when a young man.[140]

Ambrose Hanckwitz's rise to fortune was due in the first place to his successful manufacture of glacial phosphorus. Tradition asserts that Hennig Brandt of

[136] Franklin, op. cit., note 131 above, p. 127.

[137] Several members of the Invisible College migrated to Oxford in about 1647 and formed an "experimental philosophicall Clubbe" which met at Tillyard's.

[138] (a) Robert G. Frank *jr*, 'The John Ward diaries: mirror of seventeenth century science and medicine', *J. Hist. Med.*, 1974, **29**: 147–179, see pp. 152, 157; (b) *idem, Harvey and the Oxford physiologists*, Berkeley, University of California Press, 1980.

[139] R. Pilkington, *Robert Boyle, father of chemistry*, London, Murray, 1959, p. 145.

[140] R. E. W. Maddison, 'Studies of the life of Robert Boyle, FRS', *Notes Rec. R. Soc. Lond.*, 1953, **10**: 159–187, pedigree p. 162.

Hamburg, in about 1668, discovered how to isolate an impure phosphorus, a secret that he carefully guarded. In spite of this, in September 1677, Dr Johann Daniel Kraft demonstrated the newly discovered element to Boyle, and gave him hints of the materials from which it had been derived. By 1680, Boyle had devised a method employing urine but, being dissatisfied with the yield, he asked his laboratory assistant Bilger to find a more successful method. In this he was forestalled by the young Hanckwitz, who not only obtained a better yield but produced a far superior end-product. Some time between the birth of his eldest son and the death of Boyle in 1691, Hanckwitz started his own laboratory in the garden of his house in Southampton Street. It soon became one of the best equipped in England, and was the resort of people of fashion as well as those with scientific leanings. Here he developed his "fire annihilator" or "water bomb" and conducted analyses of medicinal waters and earths. He also perfected a method of preparing sulphuric ether, whose properties he and Johann Sigismund Frobenius demonstrated to the Royal Society in 1730. He found it useful in the cold extraction of essential oils.

Ambrose (I) died in 1741, and the business was continued by his second and third sons, Ambrose (II) and John, who were soon in difficulties. The firm was burdened with money commitments arising from their father's will, but John's incurable extravagance was probably even more damaging. Bankruptcy ensued in 1746, but the struggling concern was allowed to work off its debts, and happily rose to considerable prominence under the guidance of Ambrose (III) of the next generation. After the death of the founder, the character of the firm seems to have changed; it was still engaged in the manufacture of chemicals, but it also prepared the pharmaceutical products of the day. On 1 July 1746, Ambrose (III) was apprenticed for eight years to James Burges, junior, citizen and apothecary, and took up the freedom of the Society thirteen years later in 1759.[141]

John Conyers, a London apothecary, conducted some of the earliest "tryalls" on phosphorus of which we have any knowledge. It was his normal practice to make a careful note in his memoranda book of the dates on which he carried out his experiments, but on this occasion he has unfortunately not done so. In his book, they lie between those of 3 October 1682 and 20 October 1690, and, as he writes of using a small slice, it would seem he had obtained his sample from Hanckwitz.[142]

Som[e] tryalls Made upon phosphor described in Mr Boyles Booke (i) I tooke the shanke of veale bones & when I had scraped ofe the skinn & moysture I rubbed a small minute slice of the phosphor upon this bone w[i]th the handle of my knife which did not at all flame, but onely now & then smoke upon knocking & bending the bone. Secondly, I took oyle of Almonds & upon browne paper 3 double I droppt it & wth a small quantity of phosphor rubbed wth my knife handle thereon it scarse made show of so much as light or smoke, the same I did then trye with butter. 3ly I rubbed a small quantity wth salt & saltarmonick wch was not improved therby, the same allso wth flower of brimston. 4ly I tryed upon paper wett with oyle of vitriol and spirit of salt & found they extinguished it so th[a]t little or no flame appeared, as allso wth Sp: Corn: Cervi as little or less & so allso wth water in like warmer wett upon browne paper, lastly I spread P. Aureos upon doubled browne paper & a minute slice of this rubbed thereon fired verry feircely & speedier then anny of the other in so much th[a]t it appeared to bee furious in its motion & speedily burnt my Ivory knife handle wth much less rubbing. I tooke of salt peeter a little & rubbed it upon the bottom of the outside of a Gallypott & wth a small modicu[m] of this phosphor quickly made an explosion like gunpowder.[143]

[141] Guildhall Library, Apothecaries' Society court minutes, MS. 8200/7, ff. 5r, 143v.
[142] Hanckwitz's phosphorus was white and solid and not the earlier dark brown sticky mass.
[143] British Library, Sloane MSS., MS. 958, f. 139r. Memoranda of John Conyers.

Our knowledge of the life and activities of the seventeenth-century apothecary is so slight that the memoranda of John Conyers, apothecary in Fleet Street, London, warrant a closer examination. From his notes, we learn that he was the son of Edward Conyers and his wife Jane Clarke, who were married in 1632 or 1633 in the former church of St Faith's. He was apprenticed to Robert Phelps, citizen and apothecary, and gained his freedom of the Company in February 1658. When he first became involved with the Royal Society is not known, and he is often confused with William Conyers MD of Oxford, who died of the plague in 1665.[144] Although the relationship was of the remotest, it is certain that the two families knew of each other. In 1672, the records relate that Mr Hooke had produced a speaking trumpet which was found to be better than the one designed by Mr Conyers; in 1679 and 1680, Conyers was propounding mathematical problems, which Mr Hooke solved by means of Signor Viviani's book which he had recently received.[145] Robert Hooke knew Conyers well and mentioned him several times in his diary. "Wednesday, May 27th 1674. At Mr Coniers, Apothecary in Fleet St. Saw some stones of his Collection and much Ebur Fossile. He gave me a peice." On Thursday 19 August 1680, he wrote, "Conier, apothecary. At Jonathans with Coniers, Ashton and Dr Wood."

Conyers published papers in the *Philosophical Transactions* on a pump and on hygroscopes. In the second half of the seventeenth century, a fresh investigation began into the age-old ideas concerning the relationship between weather and disease. Sydenham believed that the study of epidemic illness required a close observation of the weather, a study that was made easier by Boyle's experiments with barometers and other instruments such as his "statistical hygroscope". Christopher Wren urged the importance of the study of meteorology in relation to the incidence of disease in an address to the Royal Society, and it is possible that Conyers heard him on the subject.[146] In March 1675, Conyers wrote: "Here you will find som observations made touching the weather as to heat or cold, moysture & drouth which will be taken from glasses modified into Cylinders & Conexes . . . all having 3 fs of sponge put into each glass wch varies their weight from tyme to tyme as the tyme of the yeare is . . . ." He went on to relate that he had already kept a diary concerning the weather for a year and a quarter. These glasses he suspended in a cupboard with perforated base and sides, which he nicknamed the "phenix nest". He weighed them frequently and related the variations between them to their differences in shape, which he thought might affect the gathering of moisture.

He made instruments which he sometimes called thermometers and sometimes thermoscopes. They were filled with different fluids such as almond oil, spirits of wine, or "green water made from vinegar maydew, Roman vitriol and verdigrease in common water", all designated by symbols. They were calibrated, and he took great pains to ascertain at what number they were standing, and under what conditions, speculating as to why they should differ.

[144] William Conyers had an interest in chemistry and we learn from the John Ward diaries (note 138a above) that he had a furnace of his own. He was the son of William of the Walthamstow Conyers. His will is at the PRO, PCC Prob. 11–319 f. 20.

[145] R. T. Gunther, *Early science in Oxford*, 15 vols., Oxford, [for the Subscribers], 1923–67, vol. 7, pp. 403, 538, vol. 4, p. 85. His paper on the ear trumpet was published in the *Philosophical Transactions*.

[146] J. H. Cassedy, 'Medicine and the rise of statistics', in Debus (editor), op. cit., note 6 above, p. 303.

He related the weather conditions to the state of health, and on one occasion gave a dramatic example. On 24 March 1675, he noticed a sultriness in the atmosphere with a "... smoakynes & a due or moysture cleaving to the paste & painted boarded entryes ...", the sulphurous reek continued for an hour or so and the unusual warmth for longer, "... which prooved fatall for about 10 of the clock that night my verry good friend Dr Jonathan Goddard reader of the Physick lectures at Gresham colledg, he was taken ill & sodainly fell downe dead in the street as he was entering into a coach, he beinge pretty Corpulent & tall man, a Bachelour of about 5 & fifty yeares age & Mellancholly & inclineing to be Cynick who used now & then to complain of giddynes in his head; he was an excellent mathematician & phisician, sometymes to Oliver the protector."

John Conyers was convinced that the earth shrank and swelled "... one [*sic*] the superficies at least, in like manner as the wo[o]den Pannel of Deale with an Index". He listed twenty-seven observations which he thought proved his belief. He was aware of the phenomena of magnetism, electrostatics, evaporation, absorption, expansion, and fermentation, but explained them all in terms of "rarifaction and condensation". In observation No. 24, he wrote of an experiment in which a tightly stoppered empty bottle was lowered to such a depth in the sea that it shattered. This he believed was due not to "... pressure as Mr B. would have it ..." but to "... the ayre therin shrinking untill it drawed in the sydes". He knew of the new theory of "the pressure of the atmosphere which is now strongly maintained by all the world" but remained doubtful of its validity. He carried out a number of experiments which he thought "rebuked" the theory but his results were much confused by capillarity and surface tension.

His work as a pharmacist was of ever-present interest to him. In his memoranda, he referred to the making of extract rudii and drew inferences in relation to combustion; the manufacture of aloes of roses gave him the opportunity to discuss the question of the dispersal of solids in liquids and the entrapping of air, whilst the preparation of lac virginis allowed him to suggest the method by which fossils were formed. He also made notes on the tanning of leather and drew diagrams of outsize hailstones and snowflakes, but his keenest interest aside from physical chemistry was archaeology, about which he wrote at length. Living so near to the cathedral of St Paul and having such an enquiring mind, it is not surprising that he often visited the workmen at the time of the rebuilding. The discovery of Roman coins, brick, and pottery interested him greatly. He noted Samian and Castor ware and poppy-beakers and well understand the value of strata. He wrote, "I might see the Epochs or beginnings of things and in these various heighths of ground poynt & shew with my finger the Romans concernes lay deepest, then higher those of more recent or fresher conerne". The man obviously had the makings of a good archaeologist and, as Oakley has pointed out, he appears to have recognized that the hand-axe was a primitive tool.[147]

Conyers was in close contact with the enquiring and "curious" persons of his day. He often mentioned Francis Glisson, the Regius Professor of Physick at Cambridge, who lived nearby, and no wonder, because Glisson was Conyers' wife's uncle.[148] Other

[147] K. P. Oakley, *Man the tool-maker*, London, British Museum, 1963, p. 3.

[148] From Glisson's will dated 1674, it is apparent that John Conyers had borrowed £80 from him and had not repaid it. PRO, PCC, Prob. 11, 355, f. 116, proved November 1677.

well-known acquaintances were Mr Tompion the watchmaker, who borrowed Conyers' deal hygroscope for a while, and Mr Flamsteed the astronomer, who "... resolved to make one of my weather-gages ...". John Conyers' ideas on physical science were woefully confused, but he was aware of the recent developments, even if he did not agree with them or fully understand them. He manfully tried to implement the "new" philosophy by conducting experiments and evaluating their results. His profession not only allowed but actually encouraged him in his studies, and was a continual stimulus to his investigatory powers.

The apothecaries would seem to have contributed few experimentalists with leanings towards chemical theory, but in manufacture the story is rather more positive. As Clark has noted, the diaries and correspondence of scientists in the age of Newton are full of their visits to workshops, of their talks with artificers, and descriptions of industrial processes. He quotes Boyle as saying, "In many cases a trade differs from an experiment, not so much in the nature of the thing, as in its having had the luck to be applied to human use ...."[149] James Goodwin, referred to in the Annals of the College of Physicians as "Chymist and Apothecary at the end of the Hay Market", is known to have manufactured sal ammoniac and probably sal volatile and ammonium carbonate.[150] His business must have been of a considerable size, as he made a bold attempt to gain and hold a much-prized contract for the supply of drugs to the Royal African Company in the early 1720s. He thereby gained the enmity of the College, and, because he was an unincorporated apothecary, that of the Society as well.[151]

The very successful activities of the Society of Apothecaries' own laboratory should not be forgotten. The College of Physicians had established a laboratory in about 1650 under a chemist called William Johnson.[152] Johnson was a victim of the plague in 1665, and the laboratory with the other College buildings was destroyed in the fire of the following year, whereupon the physicians' interest seems to have died. The apothecaries, seeing a good opportunity, in 1671 invited the freemen of their Company to finance an elaboratory for the manufacture and sale of chemical medicines. The inaugural meeting of subscribers was held 4 January 1672. The first operator was Samuel Stringer, but his conditions of employment were so poor that he left a year later. His successor, Samuel Hull, died in November 1675, and his apprentice, Samuel Symonds, was appointed as a temporary measure. The laboratory does not seem really to have got into its stride until the appointment of a German, Nicholas Staphorst, in 1676. Production soon increased, and the following year he was in trouble for allowing sulphur fumes to be emitted from the kitchen chimney.

[149] Sir George N. Clark, 'Aspects of science in the age of Newton', *Econ. Hist.*, 1937, **3**: 362–379, see p. 371.

[150] J. Grier, *A history of pharmacy*, London, Pharmaceutical Press, 1937, p. 143.

[151] J. Bell and T. Redwood, *Historical sketch of the progress of pharmacy in Britain*, London. Pharmaceutical Society of Great Britain, 1880, pp. 21, 23; Wall, Cameron, and Underwood, op. cit., note 8 above, vol. 1, pp. 416–417. James Goodwin of St Martin-in-the-Fields gave himself this title when he took Guy Stone as his apprentice in June 1712.

[152] He became a member of the Apothecaries' Society under certain conditions, "William Johnson the chimist being a Freeman [of the City of London] desired hee may be incorporated in this Companie and is granted, and left to himself what gratuitie he will give, on his promise or security not to meddle with galenical medicines". Guildhall Library, Apothecaries Society court minutes, MS. 8200/2, f. 18r., 27 January 1653.

Sales were made to physicians, surgeons, apothecaries, and druggists, and the venture became so successful that shares were limited to £25 per member.

An idea of the size of the Society's manufacturing operations, which included those of a chemical nature, can be obtained from the responses of the master and wardens to questions by the commissioners of the Army Medical Board in 1810. They indicated that medicines could be provided for an army of 30,000 men over the course of ten days if the emergency were great, and divulged that the average amount spent by the Royal Navy (whose contract they possessed) for medicines in the five previous years was £24,917 per annum, and the figure for the East India Company, whom they also supplied, was £21,582.[153]

THE PHARMACEUTICAL WHOLESALER AND MANUFACTURER

Pharmaceutical manufacturing may be defined as the preparation of medicinals on a large scale for retail and wholesale purposes, and necessitates the invention of and experimentation with technical improvements. The seeds of the twentieth-century pharmaceutical industry were sown as early as the late seventeenth century, and by the end of the next century were in vigorous growth.

The term "proprietary medicines" or, less correctly, "patent medicines" has been applied to those for which the sole rights of manufacture were claimed by virtue of a secret formula known only to the preparers; or to medicines for which letters patent had been granted; or to those to which the preparers have affixed their names or trade marks in the hope of establishing the sole rights of presentation.[154] There is no doubt that such medicines were already on sale by the first half of the seventeenth century. In the Star Chamber case of 1634, which the College of Physicians brought against the Society of Apothecaries, one of their stated grievances was that some of their rivals had private nostrums: "Cook hath pills and a Medicine called Cooks golden Egg, And Edwards a Water called Edwards Cordiall Water, And Holland Purging bottles called Hollands Bottles."[155] The widely advertised Dr Patrick Anderson's Scots Pills and Singleton's Eye Ointment were also being produced at this time. Anderson is said to have been a Scots physician, and A. C. Wootton has traced the origin of the mercuric eye ointment to a Dr Johnson; other physicians certainly had their own nostrums, as became apparent during the pamphlet war, but apothecaries were equally, if not more, to the fore.

Thomas Bromfield, later to become master of the Society, wrote a booklet in 1679 in which he publicized his *Pilulae in omnes Morbos* (pills against all diseases). In 1624, the Statute of Monopolies gave to Parliament the privilege of granting monopolies for the manufacture of products for fourteen years, provided it deemed them advantageous to the country. Richard Stoughton, an apothecary of Southwark,[156] applied for and obtained a patent for his famous cordial elixir under

---

[153] Ibid., MS. 8200/10, 1810, "Negotiations between the commissioners of the army medical board and the master and wardens of the company of apothecaries", f. 152 *et seq.*

[154] L. G. Matthews, *History of pharmacy in Britain*, Edinburgh, E. & S. Livingstone, 1962, p. 282.

[155] Wall, Cameron, and Underwood, op. cit., note 8 above, vol. 1, p. 283.

[156] Guildhall Library, Apothecaries' Society court minutes, MS. 8200/2, f. 254. "3 Feb. 1679, Richard Stoughton, son of Richard of Surrey, yeoman . . . bound to Peter Barton for 8 years." Made free 5 April 1687. Later, he acquired the title of doctor, see MS. 8200/4, f. 414, "1 Dec. 1713. Richard Stoughton son of Dr Richard Stoughton, having done the full years with his father made free."

this Act in 1712. A common method of advertising the patent medicine was by the "unsolicited" testimonial, a method employed by John Moore, apothecary, at the Pestle & Mortar in Laurence Pountney's Lane, in the *Daily Post* of 14 July 1736. John Moore sold worm medicines and Green-sickness Powders, Byfield's Sal Volatile Oliosum, patented in 1711, at 6*d*. an ounce, and, rather surprisingly, a book called *Columbarium, an introduction to the natural history of tame pigeons*. The Huguenot emigré apothecaries also had their lines, such as Charles Angibaud, once royal apothecary to Louis XIV, who advertised in the *London Gazette* of October 1683 his "Troches, or Juyce of Liquorice of Blois".

The post-Restoration period saw an increasing interest in the waters of natural springs for medicinal purposes. For many, the sale of these waters proved a lucrative business, not least for the apothecaries of the day. In 1700, a manor court ordered, "That the spring lying by the purging well be forthwith brought to the town of Hampstead at the parish charge, and that the money profits arising therefrom be applied to easing the poor-rates . . .". An advertisement in the *Postman* of 20 April of the same year tells of one who took advantage of the facility. "Hampstead Chalybeate Waters sold by Mr. Richd. Philps, Apothecary, at the Eagle and Child in Fleet St. every morning at 3d. p.flask, and conveyed to persons at their own houses at one penny p.flask more. The flask to be returned daily."[157]

Mineral waters, such as Philps's, quickly became putrid during transportation. As it was often inconvenient and expensive for the patient to visit the source of supply, attempts were made to solve the problem. Analyses of the waters led to two possible alternatives; the solution of the known salts in ordinary water, thus making an artificial mineral water as suggested by Paracelsus, or the administration of the extracted salt itself. John Conyers would seem to have evolved a method that was a combination of the two methods. On 12 May 1679, he wrote on the flyleaf of his memorandum book, "By Mr John Conyers, apothecary at the White Lyon in Fleet Street is prepared and sold an Essence made of the mineral which giveth the virtue to Tunbridge Waters. Any soft water mixed with a little hereof becomes in nature a true Tunbridge water of great use to those who desire to spare their journey to the Wells. Mixed with Tunbridge water itself makes it so much stronger as you please. . . . Mixed with Epsom or their Purging waters makes it of the nature of Astrop water. Bottles hereof are to be had at reasonable rates with Directions."[158]

The Epsom waters mentioned were to become the centre of a bitter quarrel. Dr Nehemiah Grew MD (Leiden), FRS, and non-conformist, was a great advocate of the salt extracted from Epsom water and in 1695 published a short work in Latin, *A treatise on the nature and use of the bitter purging salt contained in Epsom water and similar water*. Being by no means averse to the pecuniary advantages of commerce, honorary fellow of the College of Physicians or not, he obtained a patent in 1698 for the extracted salts, whose principal constituent was magnesium sulphate. He obtained his salt from a spring at Acton, Middlesex, and received £1 profit for every 10 lbs. of salt sold by his agents. One of his customers, George Moult, "chymist" and FRS, sold

[157] W. Andrews, *Bygone Middlesex*, London, Hull Press, 1899, p. 185.
[158] British Library, Sloane MSS, MS. 958. See also, N. G. Coley, 'Physicians and the chemical analysis of mineral waters in eighteenth-century England', *Med. Hist.*, 1982, **26**; 123–144.

the Acton salt in his shop until he and his younger brother, Francis, discovered they could obtain the salt for themselves from a spring at Shooters Hill, Kent. They ignored Grew's patent and, partly because their source was even richer in the salt, were able to bring down the price from one shilling an ounce to threepence a pound. To add insult to injury, Francis Moult then translated Grew's treatise into English and placed it on sale in his shop to any who bought the salt.[159] This led to a furious attack from the College, which does not seem to have incommoded the brothers in any way. Despite the fact that they referred to themselves as "chymists" and traded under the sign of Glauber's Head in Watling Street, a sign often used by chemists and druggists, Francis became on 7 July 1691 a member of the Apothecaries' Society.[160]

The path from apothecary to pharmaceutical wholesaler and manufacturer can, in some cases, be followed step by step, there being no better examples than the famous firms of Corbyn, Stacey & Co., and Allen & Hanbury. The origin of the former can with certainty be traced back to 1707, when Benjamin Morris, London apothecary, took as apprentice Joseph Clutton, the son of John and Mary of Pensax, Worcestershire.[161] Ten years after he was out of his apprenticeship, Clutton, probably a new recruit to the Society of Friends, married Mary Morris, daughter of Richard, an apothecary of Rugeley, Staffordshire. Her brother, Moses, also of Rugeley, was not only an apothecary but a "chymist" as well.[162] Joseph Clutton and Benjamin Morris were in partnership by 1732, if not before, but parted company a few years later.

Clutton wrote on medical topics, and there is little doubt that he practised both pharmacy and medicine. He issued a pamphlet on Joseph Ward's patent medicines, which included an estimate that 16,380 of Ward's Pills could be made for 1*s*. 3*d*. A letter from the founder of the County Hospital, Winchester, suggests that Joseph was the originator of Clutton's Febrifuge, although the credit is usually given to his son Morris. Joseph was supplying chemicals to that hospital at the time of his death in 1743, the governors referring to him as "Mr Clutton, Chymist". He is known to have had at least six apprentices including his son, who had done only four years of his time when Joseph died. His widow continued in business with the aid of an excellent journeyman, Thomas Corbyn of Worcester, who had begun his apprenticeship with Clutton in September 1728, but had hitherto made no effort to obtain his freedom from the Society.[163] Mrs Clutton remarried in 1747, the year in which her son gained

[159] M. P. Earles, 'Cutting the tapestry', *Pharm. Hist.*, 1972, **2**: pt. 4, unpaginated.

[160] Guildhall Library, Apothecaries Society court minutes, MS. 8200/3, f. 326, "Francis Moult, apprentice of Charles Feltham having served part of his time with him and then sueing out his Indre. hath lived ever since with his brother, a Chimist, was made free." He does not appear to have been in favour with the Society as he was refused permission to be a subscriber to the new stock for the Navy in 1703, and was refused a share in the elaboratory. In 1695, George Molte [*sic*], chemist, was a partner of Thomas Wilson in the parish of St Mary Magdalene, Old Fish Street; both men were taxed on £600+ per annum. See, *London inhabitants within the walls*, 1695, reprinted by London Record Society, 1966, p. 205.

[161] For a history of the firm see, T. D. Whittet and J. G. L. Burnby, 'The firm of Corbyn and Stacey', *Pharm. J.*, 1982, **228**: 42–47.

[162] The Cluttons of Pensax were an armigerous family, and adherents of the established church. Although it would be reasonable to suppose that Benjamin Morris was related to the Morris family of Rugeley, this has not been proved, and all indications are the reverse.

[163] There seemed to be a growing belief that it was unnecessary for a journeyman to take out his freedom and that he could save his money until such time as he became a master, as witness a letter from John Newsom in 1765 to his son, who was working as an assistant to Mr Smith, apothecary of Cheapside, but

his freedom, and within two years Thomas Corbyn had become a partner.

Morris Clutton and Corbyn forsook the practice of medicine and concentrated on the trade in drugs and chemicals. Trade had already started with the American colonies in Joseph's day, and as the eighteenth century progressed, the partnership became one of the principal suppliers of drugs to America and the West Indies. The Clutton interest in the firm ceased with Morris's death in 1755, and by 1763, two new names are to be found, those of John Brown and Nicholas Marshall; neither stayed for long. Brown may have been a member of the Apothecaries' Society, but Marshall is referred to as a chemist. The pattern of things was changing, to be fully confirmed with the arrival of George Stacey (I) in 1772. The three George Staceys, and the later Beaumonts and Messers, are never termed anything other than chemist and druggist. Admittedly, Thomas Corbyn's son, John, was a member of the Society until 1843, but it is not thought that he was in any way active in the expanding wholesale and retail business.

A very similar pattern can be seen at Allen & Hanbury's. The founder of the firm was Silvanus Bevan, who leased 2 Plough Court, London, in December 1715. He had gained his freedom of the Apothecaries' Society as recently as 5 July of that year, it having been noted a week earlier in the court minutes that, "Mr Silvanus Bevan servant to Mr Mayleigh wanting six or seven months of his time paid £6 9s. and is to be freed." He was joined some years later by his younger brother, Timothy. It is written in the Society's minutes for 11 March 1731 that "Mr Timothy Bevan, who as he says has been bred an Apothecary in the country and has been some time with his brother, Mr Silvanus Bevan, a member of this Company desires his Freedom ... by Redemption; ordered that on payment of £25 and 40s. to the Garden and the usual Fees and passing an Examination, he be made free." The redemption fees were always high in the Society of Apothecaries, and may account for the fact that some apprentices sought the freedom of other companies.

In his later years, Silvanus practised as a physician and sent letters of medical interest to both the Royal Society (of which he had been elected a fellow in 1725) and Dr James Jurin. Timothy does not seem to have been interested in the practice of medicine, and when Silvanus died in 1765, the style of the firm became "Timothy Bevan and Sons, Druggists and Chymists, Plow Court". These two sons of Timothy's first marriage were not destined to promote the affairs of the drug house, as Silvanus (II) left within two years to become a banker, and Timothy (II) died in 1773. Future expansion was left to their half-brother, Joseph Gurney Bevan. Timothy stood down in favour of his youngest son in 1775, and it was at this point that the complete break was made with the firm's apothecarial origins. Joseph Bevan made no attempt to become a member of the Apothecaries' Society or even of the Grocers' Company,[164]

---

with prospects of a partnership in the near future. "You seem desirous of purchasing your freedom: at present it will cost a good deal of your money ... you need not purchase while you are [a] journeyman. ..." See J. E. Brigg, *Memorials of the families of Newsom and Brigg*, [privately printed], 1898, p. 33.

[164] Guildhall Library, Woolmen's Company court minutes, MS. 6903/3, unpaginated. "3rd. March 1789. Joseph Gurney Bevan of Plough Court, Lombard Street, London, druggist, was admitted to the Freedom of this Company by Patrimony. He paid the sum of £1." The master at this time was James Phillips, the Quaker printer of George Yard, father of William and Richard, both FRS and chemists. William Allen, druggist, obtained his freedom of the same company in October 1800 by redemption for the modest sum of £1 18s. 6d.

indeed, he joined no London company until 1789, when he was thirty-five. Why he chose the Woolmen's Company is not known, except that it was one that had close connexions with the Society of Friends. Like the Corbyns, the Bevans were deeply involved in the wholesale overseas trade.

The origins of H. O. Huskisson & Son (which after an amalgamation in 1920 became Castle Huskisson & Co.), chemical manufacturers rather than drug wholesalers, can be found in the work of an apothecary, Thomas Towers. After working in association with William Jones, chemist and druggist in Great Russell Street, Covent Garden, the poor rate accounts for St Mary le Strand show that he had set up in business in 1767 at Catherine Street. In that year, he took Samuel Towers as his apprentice and is described as a druggist; nevertheless, he was employed between 1769 and 1771 by the Overseers of the Poor as an apothecary. Although both a pre-scriber (some of his prescriptions still exist) and compounder of medicines, it seems that his inclination was towards the manufacture of those chemicals that are used in medicine. Nothing is known of his earlier years, though it is probable that he hailed from Leicestershire. The wills of Samuel Towers and his brother George, who succeeded to the little manufactory, show that they had connexions with that county; both referred to themselves as "chymists".[165]

Leicestershire can furnish us with a provincial example of the change from apothecary to manufacturer and patent medicine vendor. Richard Swinfen was established as an apothecary in Hinckley before 1760, the year in which his son Edmund was born. Later, he moved to Leicester and took his son into partnership. Edmund purchased his freedom of the town at a cost of £20 and became mayor in 1804. During the course of his career, he was variously described as a "surgeon", "druggist", "chymist", and "apothecary". On his death, Edmund bequeathed his business to his son Richard B. Swinfen, and in his will wrote that he had given him, "... the receipts and prescriptions whence all nostrums or proprietary medicines are prepared", and that he had fully instructed Richard regarding their true composition and had not told anyone else. These nostrums included Swinfen's Electuary, which was advertised in the *Leicester and Nottingham Journal* of 4 December 1773 by "Swinfen, surgeon of Hinckley". The Swinfens were a highly respected dynasty of apothecaries and druggists, training more apprentices than any other Leicester phar-macist and commanding premiums of £100 to £150.[166]

Other examples in the provinces of this transformation are to be found in Newcastle upon Tyne and Bristol. The founding father of Mawson and Proctor was John Proctor, apothecary, who opened a shop in The Side, Newcastle, in the autumn of 1768, where he was followed by his son and grandson.[167] The story of the rumbustious John Bingham Borlase, apothecary to the Bristol Infirmary, sending out Abraham

---

[165] There were Thomas Towers who were apothecaries both earlier and later at Loughborough and Lutterworth. For further details of this company see J. G. L. Burnby, 'The Towers and the Huskissons', *Pharm. J.*, 1980, **224**: 716–717.

[166] L. G. Matthews, 'Byways of pharmaceutical history, ibid., 1963, **191**: 631; J. K. Crellin, 'Leicester and 19th century provincial pharmacy', ibid., 1965, **195**: 417–418.

[167] 'Wholesaler's bicentenary', ibid., 1968, **201**: 523. The grandson, Barnard Simpson Proctor, was an examiner for the Pharmaceutical Society, 1867–69, and was appointed lecturer in pharmacy at the medical school of Durham University.

A study of the English apothecary from 1660 to 1760

Ludlow's prescriptions to be dispensed by John Till Adams is well known.[168] Adams is usually regarded as a dispensing chemist and druggist, but he was, in fact, trained as an apothecary and surgeon. His master was Thomas Benwell of Overton, Hampshire, who had only just finished his own apprenticeship with Edmund Portsmouth of nearby Whitchurch.[169] John Till Adams died in 1786, but the pharmacy was continued by his capable widow Ann until the turn of the century, when she was succeeded by her nephew William Fry.[170] William died in 1812, when he was only thirty-three, but continuity was preserved by the succession of his own apprentice, James Gibbs. Richard Ferris joined Gibbs in 1814 and the firm began to specialize in aerated waters and the manufacture of pharmaceuticals. A liquid opium preparation "Nepenthe" was one of Ferris's best-known products, and was frequently prescribed until recently.

Some thirty years ago, the company was absorbed into British Drug Houses, a firm which came into being in 1908 with the amalgamation of four organizations with roots in the eighteenth century.* The oldest component was Hearon, Squire & Francis, whose founder was a man called Kirk, an apothecary and druggist at 95 Bishopsgate Street Within. One of the originators of Davy, Hill & Co. was that larger-than-life-size character, Alexander Dalmahoy, whose business at the sign of Glauber's Head on Ludgate Hill, London, was started in 1755. Alexander's father, William, had been apprenticed to Hugh Patterson, surgeon-apothecary of Edinburgh in 1712, and at some unknown date emigrated to the south, to Southwark. By the time Alexander was apprenticed to Francis Dalby, apothecary, in January 1737, William was dead.[171a] Alexander Dalmahoy was well enough known in his own day to inspire an amusing piece of doggerel, in which it was related that he sold not only infusions and lotions, decoctions and potions, castor, camphor, and acid tartaric, but wore an enormous doctor's wig. He supplied high-quality medicine chests, a "curious smelling bottle" which he advertised as the "Bouteille de Senteur", and an "Essence de Mente [sic] Pectorale" which was still sold by his successors, A. S. Hill & Son, wholesale druggists, late in the nineteenth century.[171b]

The eighteenth-century apothecary was a man of wide-ranging interests and

[168] John Bingham Borlase, later apprentice-master of Humphry Davy, was the great-nephew of the Cornish antiquarian, Dr William Borlase, close friend of Humphry's great-uncle, Robert Davy. Borlase came from a family with leanings towards medicine and pharmacy, his cousin Henry, father Walter, and great-uncle John were all surgeons and apothecaries. W. C. Borlase, *The descent, name and arms of Borlase of Borlase in the county of Cornwall*, London, G. Bell, 1888.

[169] PRO, Inland Revenue apprenticeship records, I.R./1/26, f. 6., 1768. Benwell soon moved into Whitchurch. Thomas Pole, in his diary, refers to Thomas Benwell and Francis Riley, another ex-apprentice of Dr Edmund Portsmouth, as both being "in the Practice of Physic".

[170] Ann Fry was the daughter of William and Hannah Fry. William was a prosperous grocer of Bristol who was in partnership with Fripp as a tallow-chandler and soap-maker. Ann's brother, John Plant Fry, succeeded to their father's business, but a business letter to William Padley of Swansea shows him to have been a druggist and chemist as well. This family of Frys was not related to Joseph Fry, the apothecary who was involved in the manufacture of chocolate and porcelain. Joseph's antecedents lay in Sutton Benger, Wiltshire, and he did not arrive in Bristol until 1753, when he was given leave by the Tolzoy to practise as an apothecary on paying a fine of fifteen guineas, whilst William's family can be traced back to a soap-maker of Bristol in 1717.

* The four organizations that merged to form British Drug Houses were: Davy, Hill & Co.; Hodgkinsons, Clarke & Ward; Hearon, Squire & Francis; Barron, Harveys & Co. (G. D. Hopkinson, 'An establishment unique', *Pharm. Hist.*, 1983, **13**: 8–12, see p. 8.)

[171] (a) PRO, Inland Revenue apprenticeship records, I.R./1/42, f. 42. (b) L. G. Matthews, *The antiques of perfume*, London, G. Bell, 1973, p. 72.

52

activities, and not deterred from acting simultaneously as medical practitioner and drug manufacturer and wholesaler. In due course, a choice had to be made, and today's pharmaceutical industry owes much to the innovative spirit of those apothecaries who decided against pursuing a purely medical career.

THE PHARMACEUTICAL CHEMIST OR PHARMACIST

In England, the title "pharmacist" was not used in the seventeenth, eighteenth, or nineteenth centuries, and is still not fully accepted today. In the nineteenth and twentieth centuries, many terms – pharmaceutical chemist, dispensing chemist, and chemist and druggist – are found, not all of them completely interchangeable. The earliest example of the dual title so far found occurs in Bristol in 1714, with the phrase, ". . . widow and relict of John Nicholson, druggist and kemist".[172] A study of the Inland Revenue apprenticeship records has shown that the separate titles "druggist" and "chemist" or "chemist and druggist" were used completely indifferently by the same practitioner.[173] For purposes of discussion here, the phrase "dispensing chemist" will be used, meaning a man who dispensed physicians' prescriptions, counter-prescribed, and made "his own lines" in the back shop, so differentiating him from the purely retail chemist and druggist or owner of a drug-store.

It is usually stated that the dispensing chemists were a completely new body of men who sprang into being from nowhere in the last couple of decades of the eighteenth century.[174] This not only begs the question of their origins but is untrue. Richard Smith of Bristol in his biographical memoirs, when writing of the dispensing druggists (as he called them), said, "These people had been in existence formerly but had been extinguished or at least their candle had burnt but dimly for some years", and quoted from an advertisement of 1754. Similar advertisements can be found in London. John Toovey, druggist and chemist at the Black Lion in the Strand, stated in September 1755 that he made and sold "all Sorts of Chemical and Galenical Medicines . . . the very best French and English Hungary Waters, Lavender and Mineral Waters, Daffy's and Stoughton's Elixir etc. Wholesale and Retail. . . . Physicians Prescriptions made . . . Chests of Medicines for Gentlemen and Exportation." No mention was made of the practice of medicine, but this was not always the case. In 1743, a chemist and druggist, when advertising for an apprentice, wrote " . . . [he] may likewise be instructed in the common Practice of Physic", and a chemist in 1766 advertised in similar terms.[175] The difference between the practice of a dispensing chemist and of an apothecary was not necessarily great, the degree varying with every practitioner. Both operated a shop where drugs, compound preparations, and household commodities were sold, both dispensed prescriptions and counter-prescribed, both made galenicals and complex preparations, both carried out in their shops minor surgical operations such as drawing teeth, lancing boils, or bandaging wounds. The major difference was

[172] Bristol Archives Office, Bristol Apprentice books.
[173] Burnby, op. cit., note 31 above, see p. 164 and tables.
[174] E. Harrison, *Remarks on the ineffectiuve state of the practice of physic in Great Britain*, London, Bickerstaff, 1806, p. 14; John Mason Good, *The history of medicine so far as it relates to the profession of the apothecary*, 2nd ed., London, General Pharmaceutic Association, 1796, pp. 47, 48; R. M. Kerrison, *An inquiry into the present state of the medical profession in England*, London, Longman, 1814, p. 40.
[175] 'The title of chemist and druggist', *Chem. Drugg.*, 1926, **105**: 100, 95, 97.

that the apothecary travelled to the patient's house, at first to supply and administer the physicians' prescribed medicines, and later as the medical adviser of first instance. The dispensing chemist seems not to have left his shop. The father of John Flint South, the surgeon of St Thomas's Hospital, was a highly respected druggist in Southwark High Street. South relates that his father had been an excellent counter-prescriber, being particularly successful with children and babies; many times he was urged to "go apothecary" and make outdoor visits, but he preferred to stay behind his own counter.[176]

It has been suggested that the druggist was originally purely a wholesaler.[177] Charters dating from the reigns of Henry VI and James II placed the jurisdiction of the druggists under the Grocers' Company of London, and it remained with that guild after the separation of the apothecaries. An examination of the careers of the Bromfield family is instructive on this point. Thomas Bromfield (I) (1643–1711) was an apothecary who rose to become master of the London company. He wrote papers on scurvy, anaemia, dropsy, and intestinal worms, and introduced his "Pilulae in Omnes Morbos" which, in time, came to be known as Bromfield's Pills. He had one son, Thomas (II), by his first marriage (to Rebecca Girle), and three sons, Edward, William, and Thomas (III), by that to Bridget, the daughter of Sir Thomas Witherley MD. Thomas (II) became a druggist after apprenticeship to Philip Scarth, a druggist member of the Grocers' Company. In due course, Thomas became Scarth's son-in-law, but probably did not succeed to the business, for Scarth's son Philip junior was also a freeman of the Grocers' Company.[178]

Some idea of what these men traded in can be gained from the inventory in 1721 of Thomas (II)'s house in Dove Court, where he stored coffee, black pepper, oyster shell, and cinchona bark, and from Scarth's accounts with Messrs. Estwick and Conyngesby of the Feathers, West Smithfield. In 1674, Scarth was paid £4 3s. 4d. for supplying them with precipitate, and they, in return, sold him lapis tutie and large quantities of rhubarb. The Chancery Masters' Exhibits describe the concern at the Feathers as that of an apothecary, but "wholesale and retail druggist" is more exact.[179] The account books, with some gaps, cover the years 1651 to 1685. The sums of money handled were large, such as £144 15s. 6d. for cardamoms, £45 for ginger, or £40 5s. for musk, and the total value of the goods in 1661 ran to £1,106 13s. 8d.

Six men, Thomas Weld, Humphrey Jenner, William Hills, Richard Turgis, John Wright, and William Marston, in 1651 had formed a "co-partnership", whose day-to-day business was in the hands of Francis Estwick and John Conyngesby. It can be seen from the first year's trading accounts that they were actively engaged in wholesale trade. Every few weeks, Estwick and Conyngesby carried out a rough and simple piece

[176] C. L. Feltoe (editor), *Memorials of J. F. South*, London, Murray, 1884, p. 2.
[177] R. S. Roberts, 'The early history of the import of drugs into Britain', in Poynter (editor), op. cit.,, note 1 above, p. 171.
[178] This family covered a wide professional spectrum, including druggists, apothecaries, a physician, a surgeon of note, and a barrister. For further discussion, see J. G. L. Burnby and T. D. Whittet, *Plague, pills and surgery, the story of the Bromfields*, Edmonton Hundred Historical Society, Occasional Paper no. 31, 1975.
[179] PRO, Chancery Master's exhibits, MSS. C. 104/130 and 131. A view which is confirmed by a will in the Commissary Court, that of a young man called John Conyngesby, who calls his uncle of the same name, "citizen and druggist".

of book-keeping. On the right-hand page were listed all payments, even the smallest, such as 1*s*. 6*d*. to the carman or 2*d*. for a bottle, and the left-hand page bore all the receipts. Payments were usually considerably less than receipts, so that a healthy balance was left. Amongst the receipts, usually the last item, was the entry, "Rec'd out of the Counter". The sums varied from £10 to over £40. Clearly, the Feathers had a retail side as well as a wholesale, but whether sales were made only to the trade or to the public at large is not apparent. The goods of the partnership travelled beyond the confines of London, going as far as Uttoxeter and Welshpool. There were no references to prescriptions, counter-prescribing, or medical treatment. The annual stocktaking shows them to have had a very wide range of vegetable drugs, a few of animal origin, and considerably more of chemicals and minerals. They also stocked ivory glister pipes and those of less exotic material; they had small and large syringes, but no surgical instruments. The only apparatus noted was a brass mortar worth £7 and a copper bottle valued at £1. They had only small quantities of the favourite compound preparations of the day, for example, crocus metallorum, mithridate or London treacle, which suggests there was no dispensary or laboratory for the compounding of the complicated recipes of the London Pharmacopoeia.

It is useful to make a comparison with the chemist and druggist's business of William Jones, which flourished some eighty years later.[180] He started to trade in 1746 in Little Russell Street, Covent Garden, and moved to Great Russell Street ten years later. It is obvious from the large number of prescriptions still extant that he was a dispensing chemist as well as a wholesale druggist in a considerable way. He supplied apothecaries, surgeons, and hospitals all over the Midlands and the West Country, yet he had a retail business from which he sold such domestic remedies as 4 oz. of senna for 10*d*., or 3*d*.-worth of carmine to the players in the nearby theatres. He had a well-equipped laboratory with still, worm, and furnace. Watson points out that Jones, like other merchants of substance and reputation, was entrusted with the collection and holding of drafts, which were the usual means of paying accounts at a distance. "Some were for goods supplied by him but a substantial part of them were held by him as reserve funds to be used as directed by the customer for future disbursement on their behalf. . . . His banking activities were a very considerable part of his business . . . and included the handling of executor and trustee accounts and the investing of surplus funds in government securities. . . ." He handled 3% India Bonds for his customers, supplied the ever-popular lottery tickets, and fire insurance, and paid their stamp duty, land tax, and poor rate for them. The practice of medicine seems to have played only a small part in his business, but from 1761 to 1766 he did have a partner, Thomas Towers, an apothecary who prescribed medicines and treatment and made postal diagnosis.[181] It is doubtful that the type of business found at the Red Cross in Great Russell Street would have developed from that of the Feathers, Smithfield.

Following the lead of Bell and Redwood's *Progress of pharmacy* (1880), many have stated that the origins of dispensing chemists can be found in those dispensers

[180] G. M. Watson, 'Some eighteenth century trading accounts', in Poynter (editor), op. cit., note 1 above, pp. 45–77.

[181] It is thought that Thomas Towers later forsook medicine and founded a manufacturing drug firm. See Burnby, op. cit., note 165 above, pp. 716–717.

employed by the physicians in their three dispensaries in the cities of London and Westminster.[182] The number involved, however, was small and could not possibly account for all the dispensing chemists of the two cities, to say nothing of those in the provinces. From the petition laid before Parliament for the proposed Act of 1748, it is apparent that both the apothecaries and the "elaboratories" springing up in increasing numbers played a part. One witness, Edmund Stallard, related that he had served an apprenticeship to a "regular apothecary" in London, and then he had acted as an operator, first to a Mr Midgley, a chemist, and then to a Mr Hall, a druggist.[183] This, he explained, meant that he had become a compounder of medicines. Later, he became a partner in the chemical business. Another witness, John Horridge, told the committee that he too had served his apprenticeship with an apothecary, and that he was currently engaged in that capacity, but earlier, before he had set up for himself, he had been an operator at an elaboratory.

The foundations of many old-established pharmacies can be found to be in apothecaries' shops. According to family tradition, Raggs of Edmonton, Middlesex, started in an apothecary's shop on the Green in 1839, and Mackereth's of Ulveston, Lancashire, is claimed to have originated in the practice of an apothecary, Dr Fell, a member of the famous Fell family of Swarthmore Hall.[184] The pharmacy in the Market Place of Faversham, Kent, housed in a medieval timber-framed building, can be traced back from its 1978 owners to Thomas Joseph Thomas and his uncle, Evan Jenkins, who bought the business in 1887. Jenkins' predecessors were the Clause family, comprising Samuel Ruthbrook Clause (MPS, 1868–95), his father Thomas Clause (died 1858), and his grandfather, another Thomas (died 1820). The older Thomas was listed in the directory of 1784 as an apothecary and surgeon. The London Surgeons' Company in 1779 had pronounced him "first mate, first rate" and he served as a surgeon on the sloop *Bonetta*. There is then, unfortunately, a gap between him and a barber-surgeon, John Allen in 1700, and a practitioner of physic, George Mourton, in 1641.[185]

A rather similar pattern can be seen in the little Huntingdonshire town of Kimbolton, where Thomas Peck, apothecary, in 1776 leased a property at 1 St Andrew's Lane at a rent of £3 10s. 0d. a year and an immediate expenditure of £50 on repairs.[186] The pharmacy was hived off from medical practice in about 1830, whereupon it

[182] 'The title of chemist and druggist', op. cit., note 175 above, p. 90; E. C. Cripps, 'Pharmacy in the 18th and 19th centuries', *Pharm. J.*, 1950, **164**: 30. Bell first made the suggestion in 1842.

[183] 'Attempted legislation in 1748', *Chem. Drugg.*, 1926, **105**: 198–199. Mr Midgley was probably the Charles Midgley, son of John, a citizen and scrivener, who was bound to Francis Moult, apothecary, on 3 August 1697. He encountered some problems when he applied for his freedom in 1705, ". . . [he] not being capable to answer in Pharmacy though understanding Chymistry, to be presented to the Court of Assistants". He was freed three months later without further comment. He succeeded to Moult's business at Glauber's Head, Watling Street.

[184] C. Ragg, *Memories of Edmonton Green*, Edmonton Hundred Historical Society. Occasional Paper (O.S.) no. 2., [n.d., *c*. 1950s]. Information supplied by Mr T. B. Horrocks to Mr D. J. Greaves of Ulverston library. This Dr Fell is probably the John Fell, apothecary and surgeon, who was taking apprentices in 1769 and 1778, and of whom Sir Thomas Frankland wrote so kindly in a letter to William Curtis in 1781.

[185] F. Haley, 'The 300 year tale of a Kent pharmacy', *Chem. Drugg.*, 1978, **210**: 896; 'A Faversham pharmacy', *Counterscope*, Bayers' Professional Projects, 1962, vol. 1, p. 1.

[186] R. M. and P. A. Hall, 'Bicentenary of Kimbolton pharmacy', *Pharm. J.*, 1976, **217**: 515–516. It was the year in which Thomas Wagstaffe started training with him; it is probable that Peck had his own apprenticeship with William Bond, apothecary of Pavingham, Bedfordshire.

becomes apparent that the shop could not be supported by pharmacy alone until at least 1920. Props ranged from veterinary surgery to stationery and the sale of glass and earthenware. George Gudgen, in the later nineteenth century, carried on fierce verbal battles with the dispensing doctor opposite, but then turned more and more to auctioneering; in this century, the pharmacist has practised as both optician and dentist, and one so organized local affairs that the telephone exchange was installed in his shop.

More widely known, but unhappily no longer a pharmacy, is the firm of Cope and Taylor in Derby. According to the pharmaceutical historian, Kirkby, who had access to certain "title deeds, all of which are in safe custody", the house in the Cornmarket was built by William Franceys of Markeaton in 1648, a grazier, and let by him the following year to John Franceys of Derby, a butcher, when the building was valued at £250.[187] William died in the summer of 1664, bequeathing all his property in Derby to his elder son John, a butcher. His younger son William was to have £90, "£10 for his binding as an apprentice to some good trade such as William with the advice of his mother and friends shall make choyce, and £80 at the end of his apprenticeship in order to set himself up".[188]

William chose to be an apothecary. His master is unknown, but in due course he set himself up in his old home in the Corn Market, brother John having transferred the property to him by an indenture dated 1683.[189] The minute book of the Derby mercers' guild shows that William rose to be appointed in turn registrar, warden, and steward; he was mayor of the town for the years 1697, 1699, and 1700.[190] During his mayoralty, he was much involved in politics and was a friend and adherent of Thomas Coke of Melbourne.[191] William and his wife Elizabeth had six sons, but only the first two, William (baptized January 1675) and Henry (March 1677) grew to adulthood. The older son was sent to London in 1691 to be apprenticed to Richard Blundell, surgeon of the Barber-Surgeons' Company.[192]

The apothecary died in 1703. His son William, then practising as a surgeon in Derby, received only £100, although it is obvious that his father was a wealthy man; the rest of his estate, including shares in leadmines and waterworks, was bequeathed

---

[187] W. Kirkby, 'A 17th century Midland pharmacy, Cope and Taylor of Derby', *Pharm. J.,* 1935, **134**: 566–568. The MS. of the fair-book of Derby corroborates that William and John Franceys were trading as butchers at the fair between 1646 and 1654.

[188] Lichfield Record Office, will of William Franceys of Derby, butcher, proved 10 September 1664. He appears to have been illiterate, and his seal was a simple W.F.

[189] Kirkby, op. cit., note 187 above, p. 566. Kirkby did not make use of either wills or parish registers and has confused the numerous members of the Franceys family. He believed the apothecary, who was baptized in February 1650, to be the son of John the butcher and not William.

[190] H. A. Bemrose, 'Derby Company of Mercers', *Derbyshire Archaeol. J.,* 1893, **15**; 113–160, see pp. 159, 155, 153; on 1 March 1692, William Franceys, apothecary, was authorized to pay £40 to the mayor and burgesses for the new waterworks being built by George Serocold, who had married William's niece Mary in December 1684.

[191] Hist. MSS. Comm., 12th report, London, 1888, *Cowper MSS.*, vol. 2, p. 413; ibid, vol. 3, p. 157.

[192] Guildhall Library, Barber-Surgeons' Company records, bindings, MS. 5266/2, f. 289. William did not claim his freedom but returned to Derby. On 14 January 1702, Robert Hardinge wrote to Thomas Coke, "Mr Gray is ill of a swelling in his mouth, suspected kin to a cancer; William Franceys, Junior his Surgeon." William, the surgeon, was buried at All Saints, Derby, on 27 April 1712. Administration was granted to his brother Henry, apothecary; his whole estate amounted to £102, of which £36 was accounted for by "The Horses".

to Henry.[193] Henry, an apothecary like his father, became well known for the magnificence of his home, his entertainment, and the high social status of his friends. Notoriety was thrust upon him in 1745, when he had to lodge Lord and Lady Ogilvie and Mr and Mrs Murray, members of the Young Pretender's retinue. Franceys was elected an alderman in 1733 and mayor in September 1747, but he died during his year of office.[194] Kirkby stated that the apothecary's practice was then carried on by Henry's son George for the next four years when it came into the possession of Francis Meynell, surgeon, and Theophilus Brown[e], apothecary.[195]

Francis Meynell, scion of a county family, after education at Derby Grammar School, had been apprenticed in 1719 to John Holmes of Derby, an apothecary, which designation Meynell used himself when he took Edmund Brown as his apprentice in 1745. It is likely that Meynell and Brown had been long-time associates of Franceys.

By 1763, Meynell was on his own, and the following year, A. Stevenson, druggist, was in possession. Francis had a son, John, who had been apprenticed to a Derby surgeon, Henry Tatem, but he appears to have struck off on his own. Stevenson reigned alone for twelve years, but then a J. Beridge, doctor, was taken into partnership. He is thought to have been John Berridge MB (Oxon.), who appears in the 1779 *Medical Register.* In the nineteenth century, W. Stevenson, dispensing chemist, was the owner.

The career of Theophilus Browne, one-time partner of Francis Meynell, is also of interest. In newspaper advertisements of 1740 and 1743, when he is located at the Market Head, he called himself either druggist and apothecary, or else druggist; there is no suggestion that he practised medicine. Whilst still in association with Meynell, he combined with another apothecary, Robert Winfield, in nearby Irongate, Derby, where a pattern similar to that of the Cornmarket practice developed.[196] On Winfield's death in 1776, Browne was on his own until he was succeeded by his son Henry ten years later. Henry, in turn, was succeeded by his apprentice, Richard Jones. Jones was the son of the Reverend Hugh Jones of Burton-on-Trent, and the indentures, which still exist and were signed in 1802, show that for the consideration of £100 Henry Browne agreed to teach him the "art of a Chemist and Druggist and Apothecary".[197] George A. Hewitt, Jones's successor in 1850, was a dispensing chemist with no pretensions to medical practice other than counter-prescribing.

[193] Lichfield Record Office, will of William Franceys, apothecary of Derby, proved 11 October 1703. In it he states that he has ". . . a one third part of the Waterworks at Leeds", which were built by Serocold in 1694. William's inventory came to a total of £791 9s. 6d., of which "Druggs" comprised £300. Unlike his father, he used the Franceys family arms on his seal.

[194] Contrary to what has been written by Kirkby and others, including the writer on an earlier occasion, Henry Franceys did not proceed to Emmanuel College, Cambridge, and there obtain an MA in 1713, in which year he would have been thirty-seven. The Derby poll list for 1727 shows a Mr Henry Franceys, clerk, who voted, and another Mr Henry Franceys, apothecary, who did not vote.

[195] This statement is incorrect. Henry Franceys had no son and the property had to revert to his father's brother's male heirs, the eldest of whom was a George Francys who was not an apothecary.

[196] Robert Winfield had been apprenticed to Henry Holmes, apothecary, in 1729, and is thought to have taken over his practice on Holmes's death. Holmes was at Derby Grammar School, and then went for a year's training from July 1718 with John Beaumont, apothecary of St Paul's, Covent Garden. He was probably the son of Henry Holmes, apothecary, mayor of Derby in 1694.

[197] E. Sample, 'Henry Monkhouse, chemist of Derby', *Derbys. Countryside,* 1972, **37**: 72–73. Henry Browne was mayor of Derby twice and was the first man in that town to light his house with gas, which he had manufactured himself.

The apothecary as progenitor

An advertisement in the *Newcastle Chronicle* of 24 November 1821 clearly shows that a pharmacy could and often did change hands between the various branches of medical practice.

To Surgeons, Apothecaries and Druggists.

To be disposed of by a surgeon and apothecary: a good retail business, stock and fixtures: the returns have been gradually and materially increasing for several years and are at present very good with a Prospect of Improvement.

Continuity of training between apothecary and druggist can be detected by examining the apprenticeship records of both Chester and Bristol. A study of the records of the Company of Mercers, Ironmongers, Apothecaries and Grocers of Chester, the city registers for the binding of apprentices and the granting of freedoms of that city, as well as the Inland Revenue apprenticeship records allows one to make "strings" of successive apprenticeships covering as many as 150 years.[198] One such string shows that the druggist of the late eighteenth century was a direct descendant of the apothecary of the seventeenth.

I. John Goulborne: apothecary of Restoration Chester who trained at least four apprentices between the years 1670 and 1687, including –

II. John Sudlow: he had two apprentices, one in 1677, and in 1674 –

III. Francis Touchett: on 27 February he became the master of –

IV. Ralph Brown: who started training Thomas Davis in 1710, and in 1703 took on –

V. Peter Ellames: one of his earlier apprentices was Thomas Rowe in 1722, and up to this point all masters were termed apothecaries but when Ellames became the master of Edward Storer of Nottingham, the description was apothecary and druggist. Both Ellames' sons, Peter the younger and Pattison, on receiving their freedoms of the city were called druggists.

VI. Pattison Ellames: he had two apprentices, Thomas Meacock and John Dyson; on both occasions, 1771 and 1777, he was termed druggist.

At least one other apothecary in Chester preferred to adhere to the pharmaceutical side of his profession. Nathaniel Basnett, apothecary, took as apprentice Robert Anderson for nine years from 1672, who, in turn, became the master of Samuel Hinton for eight years from 1682. Samuel, in his old age, had as an apprentice Matthew Hinton, who, when he gained his freedom of Chester on 30 December 1730 six years later was entitled apothecary, but when he ran foul of the Assembly in 1767 was referred to as a druggist. On 26 March, that body read a petition which alleged that Matthew Hinton, druggist, had projected his shop window in Lower Bridge Street to the annoyance of passersby and contrary to a recent Assembly order. He was ordered to take down or reduce the windows within one month, or the treasurers would have them removed.[199]

The civic records of Bristol give a similar picture of the continuity between druggists and apothecaries.[200]

---

[198] The records of the Company of Mercers, Ironmongers, Apothecaries and Grocers of Chester were held in 1980 by Mr G. H. Parry, former president of the Freemen and Gilds of Chester; Chester City Record Office, MS. M/AP/B1; J. H. E. Bennett (editor), *The rolls of the freemen of Chester, part II, 1700–1805*, Lancashire and Cheshire Record Society, 1908, vol. 55.

[199] Chester City Record Office, MS. AB/4/, f. 246v.

[200] Bristol Archives Office, Bristol apprentice books, Bristol burgess books.

I.	William Dale:	"appoticary" on 11 October 1591 took Abraham son of John Edwards of Axebridge, Somerset, as an apprentice.
II.	Abraham Edwards:	trained his own son, Abraham, William Vaughan, and Beavis Mathews, who gained his burgess status in 1636.
III.	Beavis Mathews:	his apprentices included –
IV.	John Sessill (or Cecil):	who became a burgess in 1648. He had at least two apprentices of whom one was –
V.	Richard Millecha[m]p:	a burgess in 1658, he had five apprentices including –
VI.	Richard Noblett:	Like all his predecessors he was an apothecary; he had five apprentices in the early years of the eighteenth century. He died in 1721 or 1722, but his widow decided to continue the practice and to take apprentices.

VII. Elizabeth Noblett, widow and relict of Richard Noblett, druggist, deceased:
Her apprentice, Thomas Hudson, started his service on 17 November 1722. All previous apprentices were admitted burgesses as apothecaries; Hudson's admission has not been found, possibly he returned to his home, Malmesbury.

Equally informative is the line of succession beginning with James Freeman, apothecary, who gained his burgess status in 1676 as a result of his father being a milliner of Bristol. The line of apprentices may be shown thus:

I.	James Freeman:	
II.	Ebenezer Burdock:	burgess 1701
III.	William Morgan:	burgess 1717
IV.	Nicholas Lodge:	burgess 1725
V.	Samuel Smith:	burgess 1739. Up to this point, all masters were termed apothecaries, but when Smith gained his freedom his master, Nicholas Lodge, was termed "wholesale apothecary and druggist".
VI.	Harry Farr Yeatman:	became burgess in 1751 but not in virtue of his apprenticeship started on 2 May 1745 with Samuel Smith, apothecary and druggist, but because of his marriage with Susannah, daughter of Rice Charlton, apothecary of Bristol.

Rice Charlton, apprentice of Charles Gresley, a well-known Bristol apothecary, trained at least eleven young men. All those who stayed on in Bristol to practise were registered in the burgess books as apothecaries, including Henry Durbin (burgess 1747), but Durbin was always subsequently referred to as a chemist. This was by no means the first time in Bristol that apothecaries and chemists were linked.

The burgess books record in 1685 that "John Nicholson, chimis[t] is admitted into the liberties of this Citie for that he married Ruth Hester the daughter of John Machen, Draper, a freeman. . . ." He must have also practised as an apothecary, because three of his apprentices attained burgess status as apothecaries, and he himself is termed apothecary in the Inland Revenue records. By 1714, Nicholson was dead. His son was admitted burgess in that year as a druggist, and when his widow became the apprentice-master of Edward Dunne in December, she was described as ". . . widow and relict of John Nicholson, druggest and kemist".

In the mid-eighteenth century, the dual title of "apothecary and druggist" became increasingly common and many examples can be cited: Harry Farr Yeatman (1751) and his apprentice William Hussey (1759) both of Bristol, Thomas Smith of New Sarum (1755), and a variant with Thomas Warwick of Newcastle upon Tyne (1723) merchant, apothecary, and chymist. Presumably, these men were apothecaries who had turned to the medical field to only a limited degree and still had busy retail shops behind which there may have been a limited amount of manufacturing.

The sudden rise in numbers of dispensing chemists so apparent in the apprenticeship records of the last quarter of the eighteenth century, was the result of the apothecary's greed, according to Richard Smith.[201] The great profits of the apothecaries were due to the enormous quantities of medicines that they induced patients to swallow, either as a result of their own diagnoses and prescribing, or by "an arrangement" with an obliging physician or pure surgeon. In the 1780s, it appears that a patient's bill was less if he consulted a physician and then took his prescriptions to a dispensing chemist, than if he had only called in an apothecary. Many of the dispensing druggists that Smith names – for example, Till Adams, Alexander Sheddon, and the Tucker brothers, whose father Emanuel had been the apprentice of James Bush, apothecary of Bristol in 1724 – had been the apprentices of apothecaries.

Clearly, the apothecaries played an important part in the genesis of the dispensing chemist, but the development of the patent medicine industry, with the necessity of erecting laboratories, has so far received too little historical attention.

[201] Bristol Archives Office, MS. Bristol Infirmary, biographical memoirs by Richard Smith, vol. 2, f. 162.

IV

THE APOTHECARY AS MAN OF SCIENCE

INTRODUCTION

The development and use of rational scientific methods was well established by the mid-seventeenth century. The collection of data and the systematic arrangement of ideas, the application of mathematics and sound reasoning, and, above all, the experimental testing of hypotheses, advocated by men of the calibre of Johan Kepler (1571–1630), Galileo Galilei (1564–1642), Francis Bacon (1561–1626), and René Descartes (1596–1650) were, by the time of the Commonwealth, accepted roads to the advancement of knowledge. A new intellectual outlook had evolved, as noted by John Aubrey (1626–97) in 1671, "Till about the year 1649 'twas held a strange presumption for a man to attempt an innovation of learning".

The English apothecary was, of course, much influenced by these changes. He developed methods of inquiry and investigation, he experimented, he joined societies, he wrote to like-minded contemporaries, he published his findings, and, above all, he had the good fortune to be caught in the toils of collectors' mania, be it "curiosities" or new information. The apothecary had a particular interest in those fields that most closely impinged upon his own profession – botany, chemistry, and medicine.

Although considerable advances in the description and classification of plants and animals had been made by 1760, no great theoretical principles or "laws" of biology had been developed. It should be noted, though, that the generation of scientists arriving on the scene after 1760 was able to study an immensely richer collection of natural history specimens from distant lands, which helped towards developing new interpretations of Nature based on sounder doctrines.

The mid-century still regarded chemistry as an auxiliary of medicine and not a discipline in its own right, though some significant steps were soon to be taken. The chemistry of gases, fundamental to developing chemical thought, owed much to the quantitative methods of Joseph Black MD (1728–99) and the skilful experimental Swedish apothecary, Carl Wilhelm Scheele (1742–86). In this respect, the English apothecary made no direct and obvious contribution, but he was a part of a developing scientific community, his experiments were noticed and his papers were listened to. At his lowest assessment, he provided an audience to be convinced, a critic to be demolished, and the support and mental stimulus necessary to most intellectuals.

Medicine was, in 1760, even more fragmented than botany. Many – perhaps too many – systems and theories were enunciated, some of which were fanciful and far from useful, though Albrecht von Haller's (1708–77) *Physiology* indicated the path to be followed. Clinical medicine was, however, making strides in the right direction, and here the English apothecary, with his bedside observation and daily supervision of the patient, came into his own. Whether he stayed an apothecary all his life, or elevated himself to physician's rank early or late in his career, the powers of observation, medical, botanical, chemical, or pharmaceutical, that he had learned stood him in good stead.

BOTANY

In no field of the developing sciences did the English apothecary have a better record than in that of botany, individually or corporately. It has been suggested that it was at the behest of the Society of Apothecaries that Thomas Johnson (*c.* 1604–44) enlarged and amended John Gerard's *Herball*, but, apart from its organized herborizing days, the apothecaries' first known corporate venture was the establishment of a physic garden at Chelsea in 1676.[202]

In 1680, that controversial figure, John Watts, was appointed superintendent at his own suggestion;[203] not, however, without opposition. Even though his appointment had been confirmed by the court (27 February 1680), a Mr Johnson was still grumbling that he, "... desired to know what is wanting in the garden that this great charge must be brought upon the company when 1,200 plants are there in a good condition and a flourishing garden."[204] Others had voiced their doubts by saying, "Mr Watts might be a botanick but knowed not how much a gardener." The Society's minutes until this time give the impression that the garden had been run more as a commercial herb market than a place where the study of botany would be advanced. In October 1678, it had been agreed to plant "... nectarines of all sorts, peaches apricocks, cherryes and plums of several sorts...", and in August 1679 it was reported that, "... the Company will have a very good crop of sage, rue, pennyroyal and sweet majoram and scurvy grass the next year."

There is little doubt that John Watts' energy and enthusiasm changed this garden until it became one of the most renowned in Europe. Watts' enthusiasm was so great that he was a considerable financial embarrassment to the Company; neither was he without an eye to the main chance. Within a month of his appointment, Mr Phelps in court had moved, "... that a greenhouse is very convenient in the garden" and a sub-committee was set up. A greenhouse with a stove was erected not far from the river at a cost of £138. The garden now began to have many famous visitors. In the autumn of 1682, Dr Paul Hermann (1646–95), professor of botany at Leiden, came over, and suggested that exchange visits should be made; a suggestion taken up by Watts. Hans Sloane was a constant visitor, and wrote of the exotics he had seen, aloes and crimson amaranthus. John Evelyn was equally impressed by the "... collection of innumerable rarities particularly... the tree bearing Jesuit's bark." He also described the greenhouse, "... the ingenious subterranean heat, conveyed by a stove under the conservatory all vaulted with brick so that he has the doors and windows open in the hardest frosts, secluding only snow." It is the first mention of the use of indirect methods of underfloor heating being used in a greenhouse, but, when so uneconomically run, no wonder the worried apothecaries wrote in December 1682, "Mr Watts was here and desires to have money paid constantly". After several years of charge and counter-charge, the Company and Watts parted around 1690.[205]

---

[202] R. H. Jeffers, *The friends of John Gerard*, Falls Village, Conn., Herb Grower Press, 1967, p. 91.

[203] Guildhall Library, Apothecaries' Society court minutes, MS. 8200/2, f. 253v.

[204] There are no further references to the displaced Mr Pratt in the Society records, but it seems likely he went as gardener to Sir Thomas Willughby, the son of John Ray's benefactor. See a letter from Ray to Sloane, 8 January 1689, in E. Lankester (editor), *The correspondence of John Ray*, London, Ray Society, 1848, p. 210.

[205] Unlike Pratt, Watts was an apothecary and a member of the London company. For further details of

Evidence that Watts was indeed a "botanick" and not only a gardener comes from a "curious observation" that Edmund Halley, then clerk to the Royal Society, received from him, which shows that Watts had noted the necessity of sunlight to green plants.[206]

The garden became a greater problem to the Society. For a period, James Doody managed it, something that pleased John Ray. He wrote to Aubrey, "I doubt not that he will answer the expectation men have of him and promote Botanicks."[207] Doody's particular interest lay with cryptogams. After his death in 1706, a not-too-successful joint stock company was set up and the whole project might well have collapsed if it had not been for the timely help of Sir Hans Sloane. During these years, the two moving spirits were Isaac Rand (see p. 80) and, more important, James Petiver, a man of great energy.

James Petiver (1663–1718), like John Watts, Samuel Doody, and James Sherard, came from the Midlands, although his rich uncle, Richard Elborowe, held considerable property in North and South Mimms, Hertfordshire and Middlesex. After apprenticeship with Charles Feltham, apothecary to St Bartholomew's Hospital (a not too happy choice as Feltham was fined £6 13s. 4d. for bad mithridate, ther, lond., and ther. andr.), he started on his own in Aldersgate Street near Long Lane at the sign of the White Cross. In 1695, he was elected FRS, the same year as he became apothecary to the Charterhouse.[208]

His interests were not confined to botany but ranged through the full gamut of natural history; he delighted in shells, insects, and fossils, and collected preserved reptiles, animals, and mammalian skins. He had an extensive museum of between five and six thousand plants. Unhappily, Petiver was so busy amassing his collection, he had little time to spend on conservation, and Sloane was grievously disappointed when he obtained it. No man was more assiduous in promoting the study of natural history. In an announcement of the publication of the first part of his *Musei Petiveriani,* he entreated all who travelled abroad to make collections for him. At his shop, like that of his contemporary, John Haughton, there met men interested in extending the boundaries of knowledge.[209] The White Cross was familiar to shipmasters, merchants, planters, surgeons, consuls, and apothecaries. From there, he sent a continuous stream of letters and parcels, containing drugs and directions for treatment, newssheets, recently printed books such as John Ray's, paper for pressing and drying plants, wide-mouthed bottles for pickling snakes, and, perhaps most important of all, detailed instructions on how to collect the curiosities. The botanical instructions often included samples of mounted plants and, as a guide, Petiver's *Ray's method of English plants illustrated.* He used a number of goads to spur his collectors to greater activity; he stressed the benefit to science and mankind that would accrue and that a collector of distinction could gain promotion. He was unfailing in giving the collectors

his career, see J. Burnby and A. E. Robinson, *And they blew exceeding fine; Robert Uvedale, 1642–1722,* Enfield, Edmonton Hundred Historical Society, 1976, pp. 16–17.

[206] C. A. Ronan, *Edmond Halley, genius in eclipse,* London, Macdonald, 1970, p. 95.

[207] R. W. T. Gunther (editor), *Further correspondence of John Ray,* London, Ray Society, 1928, pp. 175–176, 24 August 1692.

[208] *DNB,* vol. 45, pp. 85–86.

[209] John Haughton or Houghton (1645–1705), the first apothecary to combine his profession with journalism; he was keenly interested in promoting agriculture.

their fair share of publicity and the articles in the *Philosophical Transactions* are full of their names. Some of his collectors seem to have had also free medical advice and medicine.[210]

Ray gratefully acknowledged Petiver's assistance when he contributed many of the descriptions of the new plants that were arriving from China, Africa, and India. Ray considered him to be "the best skilled in oriental and indeed in all exotick plants of any man I know . . .; and a man of the greatest correspondence of any in England as to these matters."[211] The Apothecaries' Society were wise to appoint him demonstrator at Chelsea after the death of Doody.

Petiver was a prolific writer. His first catalogue was issued in ten parts and his *Gazophylacium* in five; it contained a hundred plates and included descriptions of plants from the Alps, the Cape, and America. He wrote a number of herbals, including *Hortus Peruvianus medicinalis: or the South Sea herbal*. Typically, he endeavoured to publish a popular journal, *Monthly Miscellany . . .* , but it failed, and the third volume was never completed. As with all such busy communicators, his works were of uneven merit, but their main purpose, which was to stimulate and further the study of natural history, was achieved. His most original work was to produce "exsiccatae" or sets of dried plants with printed labels. Labels were also produced separately, printed on one side of the paper only, and were intended to be used for labelling specimens in home-produced herbaria. He introduced three sets, Hortus siccus chirurgicus, Hortus siccus pharmaceuticus, and Botanicum Anglicum.[212]

It has been said that he was slipshod, but he could certainly work to a high standard of care, as witness his report on rare flowers in gardens around London in the summer of 1714.[213] The Valentinia knotgrass was given its English and Latin names and all the synonyms to be found in the botanical works of Ray, Clusius, Parkinson, Caspar Bauhin, and Chabreus, together with the exact references of the descriptions and illustrations in existence; in the case of "Arch. Angelica" there were no less than fifteen authorities cited. In other entries, he noted whether a cited figure agreed well with the actual plant, for example, in the case of Pona's pine-leaved Candy knapweed, he wrote, "Dr Plukenet's Figure (which he took from Sir George Wheeler's specimen) very well agrees with the Pattern which Dr Sherard sent me from Smyrna A.D. 1705. Prosper Alpinus's also is well cut."[214]

Amongst the Petiver papers, two names turn up frequently, those of William Sherard and Samuel Dale. Sherard's brother James was an apothecary, and administered William's trust for the founding of a chair of botany at Oxford so efficiently and faithfully that the university awarded him an MD in 1731. James Sherard was by no means a negligible botanist himself, and had a very fine garden at Eltham, Kent.

Samuel Dale (1659–1739) was another apothecary/botanist of note. Although

---

[210] British Library, Sloane MSS. MS. 4063, f. 51, letter from Starrenberg wanting more papers for drying plants; MS. 3321, f. 220, letter from James Cuninghame saying he had received copies of Petiver's 'Centuries and Tables'; MS. 3321, f. 110, letter from Edward Bulkeley requesting a "neat box for specimens" and "Mr. Raye's 3ᵈ volume of Pl.".

[211] Lankester (editor), op. cit., note 204 above, p. 403. Letter written by Ray to Petiver in 1702.

[212] P. A. Saccardo, 'Petiver's exsiccatae', *J. Botany*, 1899, **37**: 227.

[213] *Phil. Trans.*, 1714, **29**: 229, 238.

[214] Ibid., pp. 237–238.

apprenticed in London, he practised in Braintree, Essex, and never claimed his freedom. There is no doubt that he acted as both physician and apothecary because Ray, in the preface of his *Historia plantarum* (1686) alludes to him as "D. Samuel Dale, Medicus et Pharmacopaeus vicinus et familiaris noster...". Dale's *Pharmacologia* (1693) ran to three editions in his lifetime and many more after his death; it is usually regarded as the first systematic materia medica. He sent many communications to the Royal Society and to John Haughton's *Collections for the improvement of trade and industry,* and wrote a large and useful appendix to Silas Taylor's history of Harwich and Dovercourt. Like Petiver, he endeavoured to give each specimen in his collection every synonym known to him, and his descriptions are extremely detailed and accurate.

The number of apothecaries quite seriously involved in the study of botany was large, ranging from Joseph Andrews of Sudbury, Suffolk, a friend of Dale, to John Blackstone (1712–53), who wrote a catalogue of the plants of Harefield, Middlesex, to Thomas Halfhyde of Cambridge, John Wilmer of the Chelsea Physic Garden, and William Watson, better known for his work on electrostatics. Rather more note must be taken of Richard Pulteney (1730–1801).

From an early age, Pulteney evinced a keen interest in botany. He wrote in the *Gentleman's Magazine* on the "seeds of fungi" (1750), the styptic agaric (1751), poisonous plants, acacias, the use of botany in agriculture, and the feeding of cattle; and in the *Philosophical Transactions* on rare plants in Leicestershire, the sleep of plants, belladonna, and a historical memoir on lichens. He published two important works, *A general view of the life and writings of Linnaeus* (1781)[215] and his two-volume *Historical and biographical sketches of the progress of botany from its origin to the introduction of the Linnean system* (1790). Such a work as the latter had never been attempted before, Pulteney had originally intended it as an introduction to a flora Anglica, which exists only in manuscript form. It proved immensely popular and is still widely quoted.

Dr Watson put Pulteney in contact with two notable botanists of the day, John Hill (1716–75) and William Hudson (1730?–93), both of whom were at work on preparing a British flora. Hill published many botanical works, and Richard was eager to help him in his latest project, sending him notes, seeds, and specimens. He was grievously disappointed in the results. He wrote to his uncle, "I have laughed very heartily at your burlesque of Hill by calling him very properly a lillocking wretch.... I could almost wish I had never taken mine, for it will absolutely be of no use to me...."[216] For Hudson, he had the greatest respect.

William Hudson was born at the White Lion inn, Kendal, which was kept by his father. After education at Kendal Grammar School, he was apprenticed to a London

---

[215] Pulteney is always regarded as a zealous supporter of Linnaeus, and so it is interesting to note what he wrote to John Hill around 1758: "For my own part though I like the sexual scheme in as much as it is simple and the classical characters and orders easy to retain in the memory, yet I confess I have so great a regard for the Natural Classes of plants however imperfectly they be known at present that I would rather wish to have the artificial character dispensed with then the natural." From a rough collection of notes and copies of letters sent to Hill amongst the Pulteney letters, Library of the Linnean Society.

[216] Pulteney correspondence, ibid., letter to G. Tomlinson, 15 February 1757.

apothecary, George Otway.[217] Like William Watson, he gained the prize for botany that was awarded by the Apothecaries' Company, a copy of Ray's *Synopsis*. In 1757, even before he obtained his freedom from the Society, he became resident sub-librarian at the newly formed British Museum; there, he studied the collected herbaria of Hans Sloane, which enabled him to make an adaptation of the Linnean nomenclature to plants named in the Ray era. By 1762, the year when the first edition of his *Flora Anglica* appeared, Hudson was practising as an apothecary in Panton Street, the Haymarket. This publication is usually regarded as marking the establishment of Linnean ideas. From 1765 to 1771, he was "praefectus horti" at the Chelsea Physic Garden.

Coming at the end of our period are William Sole (1741–1802) and William Curtis (1746–99). Sole was born at Thetford, the eldest son of John Sole and Martha, daughter of John Rayner, banker of Ely. He was educated at the King's School in Ely, and, in 1758, was apprenticed for five years to Robert Cory, apothecary of Cambridge, to whom the *Dictionary of National Biography* has given the courtesy title of "Dr. Cory".[218] Soon after he came out of his time, he went to Bath, and, at a later date, entered into partnership with Thomas West. He travelled widely in search of British plants and had a fine garden. He wrote a flora of Bath, an account of the commonest English grasses, contributed papers to the Bath and West of England Agricultural Society, and in 1789 published his *Menthae Britannicae*. He was a correspondent of William Curtis and sent specimens to his gardens. On 1 May 1777, Sole wrote to him, "Dear Sir, I suppose you are equally distracted between Botany and Business as myself, therefore can easily account for your long silence."[219] In this he was probably wrong, because Curtis allowed little to disturb him from the pursuits that really interested him.

William Curtis, a Quaker from Alton, came from a family with a strong medical tradition; his grandfather, uncle, two brothers, and cousin were all surgeons and apothecaries. After five years' training with his grandfather, John Curtis, he came to London to spend one year with George Vaux, a member of the Surgeons' Company, and then two more with Thomas Talwin of the Apothecaries' Society. He gained his freedom in 1771, and it is usually said that he inherited Talwin's practice at that time, but an examination of Talwin's will made on 27 August 1774 shows this to be incorrect.[220] In 1771, however, Curtis started in Bermondsey his first garden for the culture of British plants, in conjunction with Thomas and Benjamin White, the brothers of Gilbert White of Selborne. This botanical garden was succeeded by a larger one at Lambeth Marsh and another at Charlton, Kent. The first number of his *Flora Londinensis* was published in May 1775, a flora which he hoped would

---

[217] Guildhall Library, Apothecaries' Society court minutes, MS. 8200/7, ff. 24, 130. He gained his freedom on 4 July 1758; *DNB*, vol. 28, p. 155.

[218] Robert Cory was the son of John Cory of Landbeach, Cambs., and was apprenticed to Hugh Trimnel, citizen and apothecary of London, a cultured man who subscribed to such books as Thomas Uvedale's, *Memoirs of Philip de Commines*.

[219] W. H. Curtis, *William Curtis, 1746–1799*, Winchester, Warren, 1941, p. 29.

[220] PRO, PCC, Prob. 11 – 1030, f. 187, April 1777. He wrote that he bequeathed to his brother John, ". . . the house in which I now dwell formerly known by the sign of the Black Swan and Harrow, but now by Number 51, situate between the parishes called St. Bennett Gracechurch and St. Leonard Eastcheap, and belonging to both parishes, in Gracechurch St. . . . ." There is no mention of William Curtis.

eventually cover the whole of Britain; it was a fine attempt, but proved a financial burden. It was followed by his *Botanical Magazine* in 1787, which, though an inferior production, became an immediate success, soon achieving a monthly sale of 3,000 copies. In this respect, he was a worthy follower of James Petiver, although an almost total failure as demonstrator at the Chelsea garden, a post he held in a disorganized fashion from January 1773 to August 1777.

The English botanist-apothecary did not produce a John Ray or a Carl Linné, not even a De Jussieu or a De Candolle, a Malpighi or a Grew, but they were excellent men of the second rank, and as communicators on a regional, national, or international basis they could scarcely be bettered.

CHEMISTRY

Since chemistry is one important component of pharmacy, it is understandable that apothecaries should not only have been drawn to it but also have contributed significantly to its development. The work of continental chemist-apothecaries was of major importance, and a very impressive list can be compiled from France, Germany, Denmark, and Sweden. Their work is all the more remarkable when it is realized that most of these apothecaries were not full-time academics but working pharmacists. Scheele and Sertürner conducted their experiments in the apothecary laboratories; Klaproth was fifty before he went to the Prussian Academy of Sciences; Caventou and Pelletier both ran pharmacies as well as being professors of pharmacy at the Paris school of pharmacy.

In England, the story was very different. The situation was so bad that the young T. N. R. Morson, when he wished to study the new and rapidly developing subject of phytochemistry in 1818, had to travel to Paris and there work in the pharmacy of L. A. Planche in the Rue de Mont Blanc. How much can justifiably be claimed for English pharmacy in the development and subsequent work of Humphry Davy (1778–1829) and W. T. Brande (1788–1866) is doubtful. Mr Edward's laboratory at the Hayle Copperhouse was far superior to that of Bingham Borlase, Davy's apprentice-master; Brande's background was at least as much Hanoverian as it was English, and it is probable that Uncle Johann Conrad's court pharmacy at Hanover was of far greater stimulus to him than that of his unsympathetic brother in London. A better case can be made for the Henry family and for William Watson.

Watson's claim to fame in his own day was principally as a botanist and physicist; nevertheless it is not totally irrelevant to discuss here his scientific contributions. He was born in 1715, and was apprenticed in London to an apothecary called Thomas Richardson in 1731.[221] Immediately he was out of his time, he set up in practice in Aldersgate Street. His interests first lay with botany, but he soon turned to the investigation of the newly discovered phenomenon of electricity. He was elected to the Royal Society in 1741, and four years later received the Copley medal for his researches, an award which was given to Benjamin Franklin for the same subject in 1753. Watson's laboratory became a fashionable resort for members of the court and

---

[221] Guildhall Library, Apothecaries' Society court minutes, MS. 8200/6 f. 61v. He was later turned over to John Lyde, warden.

In 1806, Davy firmly linked the phenomenon of electricity to chemistry, believing that chemical affinity was governed by the same laws as those that operated in electrical attraction and repulsion.

others to see his more spectacular experiments.[222]

He read some sixty-two papers to the Royal Society, which were subsequently published; about half of them were on his own speciality. He is seen to be a careful, systematic, and observant experimenter, and made such valuable, if not momentous, observations – as that electrical discharges are not affected by colour as some averred, or that an electric field can pass through glass, even through more than one glass separated from another by a considerable air gap, or that electrostatic attraction can overcome the force of gravity in light bodies. He was in close contact with the Continental experimenters, including Le Monnier and the Abbé Nollet of Paris, Professor Musschenbroek of Leiden, Mr Allamand and Professor Bose of Wittenberg, and excelled as a communicator of their researches.

He advanced along with Nollet and Bose in their belief that Du Fay's dualistic theory of two types of electricity should be replaced by the unitary one. He was generous in his praise of the significant work of others. In 1753, he summarized the recent discoveries by saying, "Since Mr Gray discovered that bodies must be insulated to communicate to them a perceptible electric virtue. . . . This thought [of placing iron bars in the sky against lightning] could not have happened but to those who had taken notice of the analogy between lightning and electricity . . . and no one could think seriously upon this analogy but since the discovery of the experiment of Leyden in 1746." He made these remarks when reading a letter from Nollet, who defended his own views and refuted Franklin's assertion that ". . . electrification of pointed bodies is a proof of lessening the matter of thunder." Watson faithfully translated his old correspondent's views, but it is obvious he was not in full agreement with him and stated that ". . . the discoveries made in the summer of 1752 . . . will make it memorable in the history of electricity."[223]

Watson was a great protagonist of the use of lightning conductors, particularly for gunpowder magazines and ships at sea. He sat on the committee set up in 1772 to decide whether a pointed or a rounded rod was the better lightning conductor; he, with Henry Cavendish and John Robertson, came down firmly for the former.[224] By this time, William Watson was no longer an apothecary. In 1757, he gained MDs from both Halle and Wittenberg universities and was disfranchized from the Society of Apothecaries when he was forty-two. Within a short time, he moved from Aldersgate to Lincoln's Inn Fields, became a licentiate of the College of Physicians after examination in 1759, and was elected fellow in 1784. Attempts are made to claim him for the physicians, but as he acted for half his professional life as an apothecary, this is not entirely reasonable.

It is interesting to note that Watson's Aldersgate practice was taken over by Timothy Lane, apothecary and FRS. It is probable that they were close friends, as he too was interested in electrical apparatus and sat on one of the committees in the famous lightning conductor controversy.[225] Lane is is better known for his experiments on the rusting of iron, in which he demonstrated the two essentials of rusting,

[222] *DNB*, vol. 60, pp. 45–47.
[223] *Phil. Trans. R. Soc. Lond.*, 1753, **48**: 201–216, see pp. 201, 210.
[224] Ibid., 1773, **68**: 66.
[225] D. W. Singer, 'Sir John Pringle and his circle', *Ann. Sci.*, 1949–50, **6**: 127–180, see p. 171.

that iron is dissolved to a colourless solution by dissolved carbon dioxide, and that this solution deposits a yellow rust on exposure to air.[226]

Of the scientific Henrys of Manchester, Thomas Henry (1734–1816) was the first. He was born in Wrexham, the son of a dancing-master and possible schoolmaster who some have thought to be the illegitimate son of Viscount Bulkeley.[227] Thomas was educated at Wrexham Grammar School and, like his younger brother, it was intended that he should study at Oxford, but family tradition says that at the last moment it was decided his father's financial resources were unequal to the expenses involved. He was apprenticed to Richard Jones, apothecary of Wrexham, for seven years from 14 December 1751.[228] Jones died within a few months and Henry became the apprentice of Henry Penny of Nether Knutsford, apothecary.[229] Penny or Pennee was the son of Robert Penny, apothecary of the same town and Clare, daughter of William Trafford Esq., of Swythamley, Staffordshire; his twin brother Edward (1714–91) was a fashionable painter, one of the foundation members of the Royal Academy of Arts and its first professor of painting. It is intriguing to see that amongst the last paintings he exhibited in 1782 were 'The Benevolent Physician' and 'The Rapacious Quack'.[230] When Thomas was out of his time, he became an assistant of Mr Malbon, an apothecary of Oxford, almost certainly either Ralph or John Malbon, who had been apprentices of Robert Penny in the 1720s.[231]

Later in life, Thomas Henry said his interest in chemistry was first aroused by reading Boerhaave's *Elementa chemiae*. According to Farrar *et al.*, ". . . Boerhaave and the dispensary were the best education in chemistry he could have had; no university could have taught him more."[232] When in Oxford, he took the opportunity of attending a course on anatomy, and what was to prove of greater monetary worth, became acquainted with an apothecary called Samuel Glass who had a small magnesia factory on Cowley Marsh. Glass made a particularly fine variety of magnesia, the secret of which Henry learnt by methods that may or may not bear inspection. Malbon offered him a partnership, but he preferred to return to Knutsford, where in 1760, he married Mary Kinsey, who is thought to have been a relative of the Pennys. Their first child was born in Knutsford in 1763, and the following year they migrated to Manchester, then on the verge of its industrial expansion.[233] He established himself in the fashionable district of St Ann's Square, and seems to have rapidly made a

[226] T. M. Lowry, *Historical introduction to chemistry*, London, Macmillan, 1926, p. 108.

[227] W. V. Farrar, K. R. Farrar, and E. L. Scott, 'The Henrys of Manchester', Part I, *Ambix*, 1973, **20**: 183–208, see p. 183*n*.

[228] PRO, Inland Revenue apprenticeship records, I.R./1/51, f. 102. Premium £31 10*s*. Jones was a well-respected apothecary and trained at least three other apprentices.

[229] Ibid., I.R./1/51, f. 230. Premium £50. The Penny family of apothecaries were well known locally. Henry trained at least four other apprentices including George Bew; and his father, Robert, five.

[230] *DNB*, vol. 44, p. 335.

[231] Op. cit., note 228 above, I.R./1/47, f. 195; I.R./1/48, f. 203. Premiums were £30 in both cases.

[232] Farrar *et al.*, op. cit., note 227 above, p. 185.

[233] Robert H. Kargon, *Science in Victorian Manchester*, Manchester University Press, 1977. Glass's magnesia still had a market many years later, as can be seen from an advertisement in the *Sheffield Iris*, 27 April 1830: "The Magnesia. Prepared from the recipe of the late Dr. Glass is the purest and most freed from saline and heterogeneous particles of any magnesia now made. Mr Delamotte last year assigned all his interest in the above property to E. Edwards, chymist, 67, St. Paul's Church yard . . . ." Glass also contributed to *Phil. Trans.*, 'Case of an uncommon dropsy from the want of a kidney . . .' (1749, **44**: 733).

success of his practice. In 1772, he began magnesia production. At first, like Glass, he made magnesium carbonate, but soon found that the oxide was even more satisfactory; weight for weight, it was more effective and, more important, did not lead to the distressing evolution of gas. He discovered also that he could produce an easily dispersible powder if he heated the carbonate in a certain fashion, which was kept a closely guarded secret. It had a tremendous vogue and was manufactured until 1933 when the firm of T. & W. Henry was sold to British Drug Houses.

Henry played a major part in the founding of the Manchester Literary and Philosophical Society in the 1770s and taught "Chemistry, with a reference to Arts and Manufacture" at the College of Arts and Sciences. He remained faithful to Boerhaave's teachings, so that his lectures had an old-fashioned air; however, he was well aware of Lavoisian theories, as he had translated Lavoisier's *Opuscules*. Later, he lectured in chemistry at the Manchester Dissenting Academy. In the midst of this busy life, he also carried out chemical research, not of any outstanding innovative value but what might be described as "sound". He was particularly concerned with the relationship of carbon dioxide to putrefaction and fermentation, but, being unaware that the activity of micro-organisms was taking place, he reached some confusing conclusions. He also carried on experiments, first in conjunction with Dr Percival, and then alone, into the interaction between "fixed air" and green plants. Their results contraverted those of Priestley, but it is probable that the differing observations were due to the fact that neither party had any conception of the role of sunshine in photosynthesis.

Henry was first and foremost a practical chemist. He became active in the important textile trade, being one of the first people in Britain to use chlorine for bleaching cottons, and developed a "milk of lime", a forerunner of bleaching powder. He was also very interested in the dyeing industry, and seems to have had a good appreciation of the action of a mordant. He had a great faith in the uses to which chemistry could be put, and continued to be interested in new theories. Almost reluctantly, probably because of his friendship with Priestley, he came to accept fully Lavoisier's "new chemistry", and, certainly by 1797, had parted company with Priestley's views. Thomas Henry was certainly no great chemist, although his son William comes nearer to being placed in that category.

The contribution of English apothecaries is by no means impressive, but Crellin has shown that British medicine and pharmacy have made significant additions to the development of chemistry in the period immediately prior to the general acceptance of professional chemists through education and the search for more uniform or new medicines.[234]

MEDICINE

Advances in medicine during the Scientific Revolution were slow when compared with those in astronomy and physics, and even botany. Thomas Sydenham seems to have been aware of this and made many references to the work of the botanists who were so active in making collections, developing acceptable terminologies and systems

---

[234] J. K. Crellin, 'The development of chemistry in Britain through medicine and pharmacy, 1700–1850', unpublished PhD thesis, London University, 1966.

based on morphology, which culminated in the achievement of John Ray. Sydenham wrote that in order to effect cures, ". . . all diseases must be reduced to definite and certain species like the phytologies of botanists", a not inapt comparison.[235]

Although the great Sydenham can by no means be claimed to have been an apothecary, he was equally no product of the conservative medical schools of the two English universities. He spent a bare year and two months at Oxford and was voted an MB by Convocation in April 1648, principally because he was a fervent supporter of the Parliamentarians. Sydenham had no patience with medical education as taught at Oxford and thought apprenticeship a far sounder method.[236]

The surgeon and apothecary, as has been noted, was the general practitioner of the day, but the future physician's first steps in medical training were as likely to be an apprenticeship to such a man as immediate admission to university. Not only was it a common and frequently preferred approach, but it produced first-class medical men like Jenner, Withering, and Fothergill. Nobody understood the importance of this practical training more than the apothecaries themselves, especially if it could be combined with some hospital experience.

Henry Lampe, an apothecary of Ulverston who died in 1711, wrote in his will, "It is my will and mind, that in case my son Ephraim Lampe when he cometh to years of discretion, incline to betake himself to ye study and practice of physic, that he bee putt betimes to a good apothecary in a country town, . . . where they have a deal of business for making up of doctors' bills and for visiting of patients, for three or four years, after which time I would have him frequent some good hospital, where hee may see and learne surgery. . . ."[237] William Watson, previously an apothecary, in a letter to Richard Pulteney in 1762, agreed that his recent appointment as physician to the Foundling Hospital would give him extra work at a time when he was already very busy, but he was glad to have the post as it would prove so useful in his son's medical education, ". . . an hospital of all places is the most proper for the instruction and observation of a young physician."[238]

John Fothergill (1712–80) was amongst the first to have apothecarial training extended by some years of university life, which was completed by attaining an MD. When he was sixteen, he was bound to Benjamin Bartlett (I) (1678–1759) of Bradford, Yorkshire, proceeded to Edinburgh in 1734 and qualified MD two years later.[239] In order to extend his experience, he planned, as he wrote to his father in June 1735, ". . . to engage in my summers work here [Edinburgh] but was not permitted. I am now thinking of spending the three ensuing months at London either in one of the best shops there or in one of the Hospitals . . . I propose to go by sea . . . [and] when I get to

[235] Franklin, op. cit., note 131 above, p. 135.

[236] K. Dewhurst, *Dr Thomas Sydenham (1624–1689)*, London, Wellcome Historical Medical Library, 1966, p. 17.

[237] A. Raistrick, *Quakers in science and industry*, Newton Abbot, David & Charles, 1950, p. 278.

[238] Linnean Society, Pulteney correspondence, letter to Richard Pulteney from William Watson, 11 December 1762.

[239] B. C. Corner and C. C. Booth (editors), *Chain of Friendship*, Cambridge, Mass., Belknap Press of Harvard Univ. Press, 1971, p. 10. Bartlett was a bookseller as well as an apothecary. Like the Fothergills and the Sutcliffes, he was a Quaker, and his home was for many years a licensed Friends' meeting-house. Besides his own son, Fothergill, and William Hillary, he trained a number of other apprentices and justified the remark of Gilbert Thompson that, "His house might be called the seminary of ingenious physicians."

London either to attend on Sil. Bevan's shop or get to be an assistant in one of the Hospitals."

After Edinburgh, John Fothergill spent some two years at St Thomas's Hospital under Dr Mead's son-in-law. No physician shows greater evidence of his early pharmaceutical training. Until the mid-eighteenth century, the formulation of emulsions was poor, egg yolk being most commonly used, which frequently caused the preparations to become rancid, and was also expensive. After his attention had been drawn by Dr Rutty of Dublin to the possibilities of mucilage of gum arabic, Fothergill and James Bogle-French, the apothecary who had succeeded to Benjamin Bartlett (II)'s practice in Red Lion Square, London, carried out a number of experiments on emulgents, and related the results to the Medical Society of Physicians in 1757; gum arabic proved the most effective, followed by quince seeds, gum tragacanth, and syrupus altheae. Fothergill had a keen interest in pharmacognosy and is credited with the introduction of the astringent gum kino. He was aware that extracts could vary in efficacy, and realized that it was important that the plant should not be gathered before it had reached its peak of medicinal activity, and that the minimum heat possible should be used in the preparation of the extract. He eschewed the complex preparations of the day, preferring to replace them with simpler but well-prepared compounds supported by a wholesome diet, moderate exercise, and fresh air.

Fothergill made no great discoveries, in fact, his work sounds rather mundane, but the beneficial effects of his common-sense approach should not be underestimated. His friend, disciple, and biographer, John Coakley Lettsom (1744–1815), had a similar medical training and outlook. He started a five-year apprenticeship in 1761 with Abraham Sutcliffe, apothecary and surgeon in Settle, Yorkshire, and then at the urging of Fothergill went as a dresser to Benjamin Cowell at St Thomas's Hospital.[240] In 1768, he travelled to Edinburgh for a few months, but graduated from Leiden the following year. A practical philanthropist, he is mainly remembered for his part in the development of three projects, the birth of the dispensary movement, the Royal Sea Bathing Hospital at Margate, and the Medical Society of London. This broadly-based medical society was established with the object of publishing papers, setting up a library, and encouraging medical innovation. All his life, Lettsom had a fond regard and respect for his old apprentice-master, a regard which he seems to have extended to other apothecaries, as he was determined that the new society should include all branches of the medical profession. Soon after its first meeting on 19 May 1773, the numbers were fixed at thirty physicians, thirty apothecaries, and thirty surgeons; all had to be qualified and none the proprietor of a nostrum. Fothergill and Lettsom were never anything else than physicians but they did not forget the lessons of their youth, gained from highly respected apothecaries.

An outstanding medical discovery of the eighteenth century was the use of foxglove in dropsy, not only for the discovery itself but because of the scientific approach to devising its dosage, preparation, and modes of administration. The discoverer was William Withering (1741–99), physician, but another whose initial medical training

---

[240] Sutcliffe was a cultured man who had a fine library and could read Latin and French with ease. He had been the apprentice of John Ecroyde, surgeon and apothecary of Kirkby Kendal. Sutcliffe had at least six other apprentices besides his own son and Lettsom.

had been with a country apothecary, in this case his father, Edmund, who practised in Wellington, Shropshire.[241] William may have been for a time with his mother's brother, Dr Brooke Hector of Lichfield, to whom, with his first tutor the Rev. Henry Wood, he dedicated his thesis. When Withering was twenty-one, he travelled to Edinburgh, where he was taught by William Cullen, Alexander Monro *secundus* and John Hope. He graduated in 1766. Like his apothecarial forebears, Withering had a keen interest in botany, something which was to serve him well in life.

The great scourge of the eighteenth century was smallpox and much effort was expended in its prevention and treatment. The story of inoculation shows periods of great enthusiasm and others when it was repudiated. The city of Salisbury imposed a ban on the procedure in 1723. Dr James Jurin, in his *An account of the success of inoculation in Great Britain for the year 1726,* claimed that only 1 in 99 of inoculated children died of smallpox as compared with 1 in 14 of those who were not, figures largely supported by Richard Mead in 1747. In 1756, the College of Physicians came out in favour of the practice, yet it was work in which the surgeons and apothecary-surgeons were primarily involved. These men were not content merely to take their fees, but often went into print, told of their experiences, and expounded their beliefs. Some were well known in the world of surgery, like William Bromfield at St George's Hospital; others were quite obscure, such as the surgeon-apothecary Benjamin Chandler (1737–86) of Canterbury, or the apothecaries John Chandler of the City (1700–80) and John Covey of Basingstoke. Their papers were of some merit and worthy of consideration along with those of men such as Dr (later Sir) George Baker, a product of Cambridge and student of William Heberden.[242]

Claude Amyand, John Ranby, and Caesar Hawkins, all royal surgeons, were well-known inoculators, but the most famous were the Sutton family and Thomas Dimsdale. The Suttons were initially country general practitioners until the father, Robert, announced in 1757 that he had developed a new, safe, and infallible method of inoculation; in eleven years he claimed to have inoculated 2,514 people with great success. He trained his two sons, Robert and Daniel, in his procedure, whereupon they moved from Debenham, Suffolk, and opened an inoculation house near Ingatestone, Essex. They refused to divulge their methods until 1796 – when it was almost too late for many to be interested – and then demanded half the receipts. Their success seems to have been based on a careful selection of patients, minimum actual inoculation and a sensible quiet regimen; also in the course of their work they had probably unwittingly obtained and carefully perpetuated an attentuated strain of virus.[243]

Like the Suttons, the Dimsdales are usually described as surgeons. They are first located in Hoddesdon, Hertfordshire, in the person of Robert Dimsdale. His elder

[241] PRO, Inland Revenue apprenticeship records, I.R./1/49, f. 248. Edmond, son of William Withers [*sic*] of ye Hill, Salop, was apprenticed to George Hector, surgeon, of Lillishall Lodge, Salop, for five years from 29 September 1730. In his turn, Edmond had at least four apprentices, including Benjamin Hector in 1768. Edmond Withering married Sarah Hector, sister of Dr Brooke Hector of Lichfield.

[242] W. Bromfield, *Thoughts arising from experience concerning . . . the smallpox*, 1767. He was the son of Thomas Bromfield MD (Oxon.) and brother to James, apothecary in Soho. B. Chandler, *An essay towards an investigation . . . of inoculation*, 1767. J. Chandler, *A discourse concerning the smallpox, occasioned by Dr Holland's essay*, 1761. J. Covey, 'Further observations & facts relative to . . . inoculation. . . .', *Lond. med. J.*, 1787. G. Baker, *An inquiry into the merits of a method of inoculating the smallpox*, 1766.

[243] D. van Zwanenberg, 'The Suttons and the business of inoculation', *Med. Hist.*, 1978, **22**: 71–82.

son, John, settled in Hertford, and both his sons are said to have had an MD.[224] A medical career was a strong tradition within the family. Robert's younger son, his namesake, an early convert to Quakerism, crossed the River Lea to practise as a surgeon in Theydon Gernon, where he was in trouble in 1663 for working without a bishop's licence. In the next generation, both his sons, John and William, also became surgeons. John took over his father's practice, and William moved to Bishop's Stortford, where he was mentioned as a surgeon in 1715. William's branch gave rise to the bankers and surgeons of Hitchin, whilst John at Theydon became the father of Thomas, the best known of the family and the most famous of all inoculators.[245]

Born in 1712, Thomas was his father's pupil until John died; he then went to study under Joshua Symonds and John Girle, surgeons of St Thomas's Hospital. He settled in Hertford, where a relative had left a high medical reputation, and became a remarkably successful inoculator. Unlike the mercenary Suttons, he published his methods for the benefit of mankind in 1767, and it can now be seen that their procedures were exceptionally similar. In 1761, when he was forty-nine Dimsdale graduated MD of King's College, Aberdeen.

From the earliest years, it was recognized that inoculation smallpox was just as contagious as natural. Dr Richard Beard of Worcester told Jurin that he would like to see the infirmary for inoculation established *outside* the town, but it is doubtful if any true isolation was enforced until the days of John Haygarth (1740–1827), physician of Chester. By the 1750s, private inoculation hospitals for the care of patients for five or six weeks, usually owned by the inoculator and under his sole jurisdiction, were established institutions. One of the earliest was that of Thomas Frewen (1704–91) of Rye, Sussex. There he practised as an apothecary and surgeon, and set up an inoculation hospital.[246] He published in 1749 his *The practice and theory of inoculation*, in which he narrated his experience of 350 cases amongst which there had been only one death. He laid great stress on the patient's constitution and tailored his preparative treatment accordingly. He advanced the theory that smallpox and many other diseases were propagated by animalcula hatched from eggs lodged in the hairs and pores of human bodies. The treatise was "latinised", and on the strength of it he received an MD from Utrecht. In 1759, he published another carefully reasoned paper in which he showed that the development of smallpox after exposure to infection could not be checked by the administration of Aethiops mineral, which had been the opinion of Boerhaave. Both Frewen and Dimsdale, on the strength of their MDs gained in middle age without any further periods of formal study, are often claimed to be physicians, but the grounds for this are flimsy.

Vaccination or deliberately induced cowpox (vaccinia) was without doubt known in the West Country in the early eighteenth century and probably in most dairying

[244] R. H. Fox, *Dr John Fothergill and his friends, chapters in eighteenth century life*, London, Macmillan 1919, p. 82. Robert Dimsdall [*sic*] was admitted pensioner at St Catherine's, Cambridge, 5 March 1679 and became MB (1684) and MD (1696). The MD of his brother, Sir John, has not been traced.

[245] William's grandson, John, was apprenticed to John Midwinter, apothecary of Hitchin in 1757.

[246] G. Miller, *The adoption of inoculation for smallpox in England and France*, Philadelphia, University of Pennsylvania Press, 1957, p. 166.

districts such as Leicestershire and Cheshire.[247] A man who is almost out of our period, Edward Jenner (1749–1823), brought it to the notice of the "establishment". It should be noted that his training in medicine was little different from many of the men mentioned above. The son of a clergyman, he was apprenticed to George Hardwicke, surgeon and apothecary of Chipping Sodbury, for seven years on 1 August 1764.[248] In 1770, he went to London to become a student of John Hunter and to listen to the lectures of George Fordyce and Thomas Denman. By the end of 1772, he had returned to Gloucestershire to practise as a general practitioner. It was not until he moved to Cheltenham in 1790 that he decided to turn physician and busied himself with pursuing a degree. He received an MD of St Andrews University on 8 July 1792, on the recommendation of J. H. Hicks MD of Gloucester and C. H. Parry MD of Bath, when he was forty-three.

Midwifery, with the notable exceptions of the Huguenot Chamberlen family, William Harvey, and his friend Percival Willughby, commanded little academic interest until the early decades of the eighteenth century. From the parish poor law accounts, it is known that the surgeons and apothecaries employed by the authorities not infrequently "laid a woman" (see p. 34), so it is no surprise that this new concern arose in the main amongst these general practitioners.

Edmond Chapman (fl. 1708–37) of Halstead, Essex, and London, and Benjamin Pugh (fl. 1738–75), of Chelmsford, both surgeons and apothecaries, were clever exponents of the use of the delivery forceps and wrote noteworthy books on midwifery. The Scotsman, William Smellie (1697–1763), who has been called "the master of British midwifery", was a surgeon and apothecary in Lanark until he came to London in 1738.[249] He did not graduate MD from Glasgow until 1745, when he was forty-seven, and thereafter continued to practise the manual art of an obstetrician. The denigrations by his detractors notwithstanding, he was a man of liberal education and culture.

The most eminent men in this field were probably Thomas Denman (1733–1815) and Charles White (1728–1813), two of the founders of the school of medical practitioners known as the English Contagionists. White, having had the drive and good fortune to found the Manchester Infirmary, became its chief surgeon at the age of twenty-four. He must be accounted a pure surgeon, though it is not out of place to mention that his father, Thomas White (1695–1776), practised as a surgeon and apothecary in Manchester, having been apprenticed to Edward Baker, a London apothecary, in 1712. Similarly, Thomas Denman was the son of an apothecary in Bakewell, Derbyshire.[250] Like Thomas White, John Denman (1693–1752) taught his

[247] The value of deliberately induced cowpox taken directly from the cow was well understood by milkers in Cheshire in the mid-1930s; vaccination by a doctor was spoken of as being a very recent development. See also, P. Razzell, *The conquest of smallpox*, Firle, Sussex, Caliban Books, 1977.

[248] D. M. Fisk and other authorities such as F. D. Drewitt say that Jenner was apprenticed to a Mr Ludlow of Chipping Sodbury, the dates varying from 1761 to 1763; this is not borne out by the Inland Revenue apprenticeship records, I.R./1/55, f. 122. It is probable that the Ludlow and Hardwicke families were closely linked.

[249] H. R. Spencer, *The history of British midwifery, from 1650 to 1800*, London, Bale & Danielsson, 1927, p. 45.

[250] John Denman came from a well-known armigerous family of Nottinghamshire, and was apprenticed to John Farrer, senior, apothecary of Mansfield in 1711; an earlier Thomas Denman of East Retford had been apprenticed to John Smyth, citizen and apothecary of London in 1657.

son the art of an apothecary. When Denman, came to London in 1754, as he wrote in his memoirs, he "... had a very competent knowledge of pharmacy and knew as much of the diseases as the frequent reading of Sydenham's works and a few other books could give."[251] After attendance at St George's Hospital and two anatomical courses, he became a Royal Navy surgeon. On leaving the navy after nine years, he attended further lectures in anatomy and midwifery, and attained his MD at Aberdeen in 1764, when he was thirty-one. Like Smellie, he continued in obstetrical work for the remainder of his long life.

The South-West produced a number of men of high calibre, men such as John Mudge (1721–93); the son of Zachariah, master of Bideford grammar school and prebendary of Exeter, he was a popular general practitioner in Plymouth. He wrote on many subjects: on the research into inoculation he had carried out with two other local apothecary-surgeons, Longworthy and Arscott of Plympton; on the lateral operation for the stone; and on the reflecting telescope; for this last work he received the Copley medal and was elected a fellow of the Royal Society in 1777. He introduced an inhaler for the relief of catarrh, which proved useful, and in 1784, when he was over sixty, he obtained an MD at King's College, Aberdeen.[252] Rather better known today is Edward Spr[e]y, principally because of the bizarre and revolting experiments he conducted on chickens and dogs in order to prove that animals and humans can survive for an appreciable number of days, eating and drinking normally, after they have swallowed liquid lead. His paper on the subject was read before the Royal Society and published in the *Transactions*. Spry was apprenticed to George Woolcombe for five years from 1 July 1742, probably of the same family as may have supplied the apprentice-master for Mudge.[253]

All these men, Mudge, the Chandlers, Frewen, and Spry, had their apprentices, to whom, one hopes, they ably passed on their experience and enthusiasm. Mudge, like Bartlett and Sutcliffe in the north of England, had a veritable training school, as did his fellow-Devonian, Nicholas Tripe of Ashburton. In 1754, Tripe carried out an unusual dissection, which, in conjunction with the well-known John Huxham, he reported to the Royal Society. A body had been found in a vault of Staverton church which, although it had been buried for eighty years, was in a remarkable state of preservation. Tripe described in detail its careful dissection, concluding that the state of the body was due to the pitch- and tar-soaked cloths in which it was wrapped, and not to any miraculous agency – a conclusion that shows a suitably dispassionate scientific approach.[254]

[251] J. Denman, *An introduction to the practice of midwifery*, 7th ed., London, 1832, preface.
[252] *DNB*, vol. 39, pp. 254–255. One of Mudge's brothers, Zachariah (1714–53), was a surgeon on an East Indiaman and died at Canton, whilst another, Thomas (1717–94), was a horologist of note. The Mudge and Cookworthy families were close friends; John Mudge was the master of William Cookworthy, nephew of the apothecary-discoverer of English porcelain of the same name.
[253] It is not known who trained John Mudge, but George, John, and Thomas Woolcomb took many apprentices between 1730 and 1783. Munk wrote of Spry that he "was destined for the church, had a good classical education and was matriculated at Oxford but soon left university, went to Plymouth and was apprenticed for five years...." (W. Munk, *Roll of the Royal College of Physicians of London*, 3 vols., London, Royal College of Physicians, 1878, vol. 2, pp. 281–283.) In this, Munk was not entirely correct. Spry received an Aberdeen MD in 1759 and a Leiden one in 1768, but did not matriculate at Exeter College, Oxford, until 12 October 1773 when he was forty-five.
[254] *Phil. Trans. R. Soc. Lond*, 1752, **47**: 253.

The contribution of the apothecary-surgeon to run-of-the-mill medical practice has been largely ignored, and still more has that to medical innovation; one might suspect that it has been deliberately played down, as Roberts has suggested.[255] If a man became a credit to his profession, then the emphasis was placed on his university life – if he went to one, or to his MD – if he attained one. Lettsom is proclaimed to have been a product of Edinburgh, yet his stay there was of only a few months' duration, whilst his time in Leiden, from whence his MD emanated, was even shorter. Rook has shown that the time students spent in Leiden was much less than has been generally believed.[256]

Fine work was carried out by men of the calibre of William Heberden the elder and Francis Glisson (both of Cambridge University), and John Huxham and Richard Mead (both of Leiden University), but the contribution of the apothecary-surgeon to advances in medicine should not be ignored. There is little doubt that apprenticeship augmented by higher study, together with an intelligent and experimental approach, was one important route to medical innovation in the eighteenth century.

[255] Roberts, op. cit., note 26 above, p. 363.
[256] A. Rook, 'Cambridge medical students at Leyden', *Med. Hist.*, 1973, **17**: 256–265, see p. 264.

V

THE EDUCATION AND CULTURAL INTERESTS
OF THE APOTHECARY

The apothecary obtained his professional training by apprenticeship, a system which, at its best, as Clark has said "... was fully justified".[257] Amongst its benefits was the direct transmission to the apprentice of a fund of clinical experience, the advantage of continuously attending the same patients and thereby seeing the progression of a disease, and a practical training that was free from the detrimental interference of both theorists and theories. This last point was not solely confined to the study of medicine. Pilkington believed that Boyle was able to demolish "the four-element system of the scholastics" and "the three-principle notion of the alchemists" because, amongst other things, "... he had not been to the university and so he escaped prolonged indoctrination with scholastic teaching ..."[258]

The Statute of Artificers (1563) made apprenticeship a legal necessity for the practice of all trades and crafts, and demanded that it should last for seven years.[259] Cameron stated that the apothecaries of the London company chose their apprentices with care and that in the time of Queen Anne their education, at least in pharmacy, was efficient.[260] A boy aged between fourteen and sixteen was taken to the Hall and there orally examined before the Private Court as to his general knowledge. The examiners laid particular stress on his ability to read and write Latin, and we know of at least one boy who was rejected for insufficiency in that subject.[261] After his time was finished, the young man was again examined by the court; most passed, but by no means all. On 10 December 1636, Arthur Denham, apprentice of Henry Field was not found "... so sufficient as is fitting for an Apothecary", but was allowed his freedom on the grounds that his master had afforded him insufficient opportunities for learning, and on condition that he keep an able journeyman to instruct him in the art.[262] Another who was granted his freedom on similar conditions was Edward Underwood. He was told he was "... to take no apprentice for two years, during

---

[257] Clark, op. cit., note 7 above, pp. 609–610.

[258] Pilkington, op. cit., note 139 above, p. 143.

[259] M. G. Davies, *The enforcement of English apprenticeship, 1563–1642*, Oxford University Press, 1971, p. 9. The Act specified the trades and crafts by name, which contributed to its undoing. The courts ruled in the seventeenth century that any trade or craft not named in the Act was not subject to it, and the Industrial Revolution created new trades in their dozens, all of them unheard of in 1563.

[260] Wall, Cameron, and Underwood, op. cit., note 8 above, vol. 1, p. 78.

[261] C. R. B. Barrett, *The history of the Society of Apothecaries of London*, London, Eliot Stock, 1905, p. 103 (6 February 1683). The London apothecaries were not the only ones to insist on a proficiency in Latin. The by-laws of the Barber-Surgeons' Company, revised in 1709 and still in force in 1745, stated that an apprentice had to pass an examination in Latin at the Hall before he could be bound. However, as this was a company of many occupations unlike the Apothecaries (see p. 15), one must doubt whether this by-law was enforced.

[262] Guildhall Library, Apothecaries' Society court minutes, MS. 8200/1, f. 360r. Field explained that he compounded few medicines himself but sold those made by other "good and approved Apothecaries". Denham probably continued to run the same type of pharmacy, as in August 1660, the year he was called to the Livery, he asked to have liberty to take two apprentices as a "grocer and apothecary" (MS. 8200/2, f. 59v.).

which tyme he shall keep an able journeyman, for that he is, both this Company and the College, found to be very ignorant in the profession of an apothecary".[263]

During his apprenticeship, the boy was taught how to dispense the complicated prescriptions of the physicians, how to compound the pharmacopoeial preparations, and recognize the drugs that were in use. From the reports of the censors who "searched" the apothecaries' shops, it is apparent that the College expected the apothecary to stock the full run of preparations in current use. The apprentice attended the Society's herborizing expeditions and lectures at the Chelsea Physic Garden. The recognition of simples was regarded as particularly important from the earliest days of the Company. As early as May 1620, it is recorded that, "Thursday after Whitsonweeke was appointed for the Simplinge Daie and the Companie to meete at Pauls at 5 in the morneinge at furthests". At first, there was only one herborizing day a year, but they gradually increased in number until there were six, at approximately monthly intervals during the summer. On 26 March 1680, it was "Ordered that there be four private herborising days this year besides the generall herbarising day and preparatory daye".[264]

The origins of the Physic Garden can be traced back to 1673 when a three-and-a-half-acre site was rented for building a barge-house – an important status symbol – and for a garden that would not only redound to the credit of the Society but was essential for the education of the apprentices. The garden for much of its early existence proved a financial problem, and at no time was it worse than when a garden committee was set up after Samuel Doody's death in 1706. Eventually in January 1708, it was decided to set up a joint stock of ninety subscribers, the moving spirits being James Petiver and Isaac Rand (see p. 64). The venture did not prove a success, probably because the aims of the garden committee and the subscribers were at complete variance, the former believing that the garden should be organized mainly for educational purposes, and the latter expecting a profit-making concern.[265]

In spite of its predicament James Petiver was appointed demonstrator in 1709, and towards the end of his life (1718) was helped by Rand. In 1724, Rand was given the new position of "praefectus horti" or director of the garden. Among other duties, he had to give at least two demonstrations in the garden in each of the six summer months and to transmit to the Royal Society the fifty specimens a year demanded by the terms of Sloane's gift.[266] After he had been in this position for six years, Rand published at the Apothecaries' expense *Index plantarum officinalium . . . in horto Chelseiano*, a work which, unlike Philip Miller's *Catalogus*, was aimed at instructing the apprentice. Rand's appointment was probably a sop to a scheme proposed by Zachariah Allen that a respository for drugs and materia medica should be established in the hall and that a lecturer should be appointed at £40 a year to give two courses of lectures annually, each six weeks long. This idea, unfortunately, was not pursued, even though it was fleetingly revived in 1748 or 1749 when John Wilmer was

[263] Ibid., MS. 8200/1, f. 452v. (11 August 1646).

[264] Ibid., MS. 8200/2, f. 256r.

[265] Wall, Cameron, and Underwood, op. cit., note 8 above, vol. 1, pp. 164, 167.

[266] As is well known, the Society's problems in relation to their physic garden were solved by the clear-headedness and generosity of Sir Hans Sloane.

made demonstrator.[267]

Apothecaries were not the only people to recognize the value of a physic garden. The College of Physicians decided to establish one in 1586, and selected John Gerard as its curator. The Company of Barber-Surgeons and Tallow-Chandlers of Newcastle upon Tyne had one as early as 1620, for amongst their disbursements is the entry: "It. paid at the Gardiners for the Companie 1s. 4d." And in 1632: "Ittem paid for dressing the garden and for seeds 17s. 4d. Ittem paid for weeding the garden 1s. 4d." After the Hall's rebuilding in 1730, it was described as having, besides a square, two other gardens for herbs, which were attended by a gardener.[268]

Two pamphlets were published in 1704, *Tentamen medicinale* (which had for part of its subtitle, '. . . wherein the latter [i.e. apothecaries] are proved capable of a skilful composition of medicines, and a rational practice of physick') and *Reasons why the apothecary may be suppos'd to understand the administration of medicines*. It was pointed out that lectures and demonstrations were to be seen at the hall of the Barber-Surgeons, the latter pamphlet observing that the anatomical dissections were open to apothecaries as well as physicians.[269] This form of instruction was not confined to London. In Salisbury, probably as early as 1613 and certainly by 1675, the Company of Barber-Surgeons and Silk-Weavers made anatomies, ". . . for the better increase of the skill and knowledge among Chirurgeons and barbers".[270] In Newcastle, the teaching of anatomy was in progress by about 1690 as the minute of 23 May 1692 shows, "Disburst about ye man that was given the Company for dissection. £4 10s. 9d.". In 1711, it was decided to send to London for a skeleton, which was not to exceed six guineas.

As Cameron has noted, the charter of the Apothecaries' Society did not require them to examine a candidate for the freedom in any subject other than pharmacy. The student seems to have been well trained in pharmaceutics and materia medica, he could probably obtain a smattering of chemistry from the Society's chemical laboratory, but for medical practice he was dependent on his own efforts, and the results of these were not subject to assessment.[271] Deficiencies could be, and should have been, made good by extensive reading. The anonymous author of the *Tentamen medicinale* said that Gibson's *Epitome* was popular, but that James Keill's work on anatomy was usually recommended, and that the books of Willis, Sydenham, Morton, Archibald Pitcairne, and Boyle were all available. Nearer to their own field were Ray's *Historia plantarum* and their fellow apothecary Samuel Dale's *Pharmacologia*.

Intensive reading was an accepted method of obtaining expertise in medicine, as witness Sir Thomas Browne's long list of books which he sent to the young Henry Power in 1646. Although the universities appear never to have urged the medical student to practical considerations, Browne was not so shortsighted. He wrote, "The knowledge of Plants, Animals and Mineral . . . may be your subsidiary study and, so

[267] Wall, Cameron, and Underwood, op. cit., note 8 above, pp. 171, 174.

[268] F. C. Pybus, 'The company of barber surgeons and tallow chandlers of Newcastle upon Tyne', *Proc. Roy. Soc. Med.*, 1928, **20–25**: 287–296, see pp. 290, 288.

[269] Since the union of the London barbers and surgeons in 1540, a board of examiners had been set up and the teaching of anatomy introduced, the company being allocated four executed felons a year.

[270] Haskins, op. cit., note 39 above, p. 367.

[271] Wall, Cameron, and Underwood, op. cit., note 8 above, vol. 1, p. 79.

far as concerns physic, is attainable in gardens, fields, Apothecaries' and Druggists' shops. . . . See what Apothecaries do. . . . See chymical operations in hospitals, private houses. . . . Be not a stranger to the useful part of Chymistry. See what Chimistators do in their officines." Power took this advice to heart, carried out chemical experiments, herbalized, and dissected dead and living dogs.[272] Thomas Wharton, in a letter to Mrs Church in May 1673 about her son James, wrote, "But now the improvement must wholly arise from himselfe . . . by his owne practise & thereupon carefully reading & extracting & constantly & exactly noting for his private use & memory what he shall read upon every disease. . . ."[273]

At a slightly later date, and with increasing frequency as time passed, surgeons held private classes in anatomy and dissection, William Cheselden, for example, began in 1711 a course of thirty-five lectures, which he repeated four times a year. As apothecaries were by no means averse to trying their hands at minor surgery, they possibly attended some of the courses set up in the first instance for budding surgeons. There are a few indications that the training of these two branches of medicine may not have been so dissimilar. It has already been noted (pp. 39–40) that a man who had been the apprentice of a member of the London Society of Apothecaries was without difficulty admitted to the freedom of the Barber-Surgeons' Company as a foreign brother. Conversely, in the 1760s, John Newsom was admitted to the Society when an assistant of Mr Smith, apothecary in Cheapside, largely on his experience as a surgeon's mate on an East Indiaman. Likewise, William Curtis, the botanist, gained his freedom not only because of the training he had received from his grandfather, an apothecary in Alton, and the two years he had passed with Thomas Talwin, a member of the Society, but because he had spent a year with George Vaux, a prominent member of the London Surgeons' Company.[274] Thus, the artificial halves of the profession were being "officially" drawn together.

Classes in chemistry, such as those of George Wilson, were also organized in London, as they were in pharmacy. John Quincy, apothecary, translator of the aphorisms of Sanctorius (for which he was awarded an MD by Edinburgh University), and author of the immensely popular *English dispensatory*, used to deliver lectures in his own house.[275]

Nevertheless, it was long before academic studies were a legal requirement, as they had been for many years in France and Germany. In 1536, a Parisian ordinance required pharmacy apprentices to attend two lectures a week on pharmacy, given by a member of the faculty of medicine. In Poitiers (1588), only those candidates who had attended lectures on the art and science of pharmacy could become masters. In the same year, the pharmacists of Montpellier established a collection of drugs and made Bernardhin Duranc, one of their members, curator, with the obligation to display and explain the whole materia medica to students three times a year.[276] At the same

[272] Robb-Smith, op. cit., note 6 above, pp. 343–345.

[273] *Lancet*, 1949, **257**: 1194–1195. Copy of Thomas Wharton's letter to Mrs Church.

[274] Brigg, op. cit., note 163 above, pp. 32–33; Guildhall Library, Apothecaries' Society court minutes, MS. 8200/8, f. 81.

[275] *DNB*, vol. 47, p. 112. Quincy died in 1722, and the following year his lectures were published by his friend Dr Peter Shaw as *Praelectiones pharmaceuticae*.

[276] E. Kremers and G. Urdang, *History of pharmacy*, 4th ed., Madison, Wis., J. B. Lippincott, 1976, p. 76. They claim Duranc was the first practising pharmacist to become officially a member of the teaching

university, a chair of surgery and pharmacy was created in 1601, and one of pharmaceutical chemistry in 1675. Many famous pharmacists, especially those with leanings towards chemistry such as Lefebvre and Lémery in the seventeenth century, and Rouelle and Baumé in the eighteenth, supplemented these courses with private ones.

Although examinations of competency were required in Germany from an early date, the first obligatory tests of a fixed course of study were not set until 1725 in Prussia. In order to be a pharmacist of the first class, the candidate had to attend a course at the Collegium Medico-Chirurgicum in Berlin, an institution which had been founded in 1718 primarily for the education of military physicians and surgeons. In Germany, as in France, private institutes were set up, such as that of J. B. Trommsdorff in Erfurt and J. C. Wiegler in Langensalza, Thuringia.[277]

London was all through the period under review the main centre of pharmaceutical, and for that matter, surgical education, a fact that was well understood at the time of the union of barbers and surgeons in 1540.[278] The bindings of both companies show that apprentices came from all over England and Wales. Many returned to practise in their own districts, and there set up dynasties of apothecaries, whilst others practised in London and, one imagines, transmitted back to their colleagues the latest developments of the capital. The standards in the provinces must have varied from the good to the abominable. It would seem only too true that the College of Physicians exercised two yardsticks, one for London and its suburbs, and another for the country. On 25 June 1694, Thomas Turberville presented himself to the College for the licentiate's examination, but failed in therapeutics; nevertheless, on promising to go to Wales and practise there for some years before practising in London, he gained his licence. Dr William Briggs (MD, oculist and physician-in-ordinary to William III), when a junior fellow, received a letter of complaint from Dr John Gostlin, the master of Caius, concerning the stupid and unskilful men licensed for country practice by the College.[279]

Many believed that any educated man could become proficient in medicine, as was written in 1652, "Yet it is easy for any scholar to attaine to such a measure of Physick as may be of use to him both for himself and others", which could be attained by seeing one dissection, reading Fernel and a herbal, and studying the native simples rather than the apothecaries' imported drugs.[280] Clergymen commonly practised medicine, either from inclination, economic necessity, as a duty to God, or because of adherence to a currently unacceptable religious belief.

John Ward had an excellent training in medicine at Oxford, largely on his own initiative, but he never took his MB, and forsook medicine for the church.[281] He did

---

staff of any European university. More than one attempt was made by the Parisian pharmacists to set up organized official academic instruction but they had to be abandoned because of opposition from the physicians; success was not fully attained until the French Revolution.

[277] Ibid., pp. 97, 428–429. The physicians of Bavaria as early as 1595 set oral, written, and practical examinations for pharmacy students.

[278] In the preamble of the Act 32 Henry VIII c. 42, particular mention is made of the importance of London surgeons in training those of the provinces.

[279] Clark, op. cit., note 7 above, pp. 518, 250*n*. It is of interest to note that the cousin of Dr Briggs's wife was the daughter of Sir Thomas Witherley MD, and married Thomas Bromfield, the apothecary.

[280] Ibid., pp. 248–249.

[281] Frank, op. cit., note 138(a) above, pp. 152–156, 159–160.

not, however, forget his earlier interests and, when at Stratford-upon-Avon, looked after not only the spiritual wellbeing of his flock but treated their bodily ailments as well. Technically, he was an empiric, but his training was no whit the worse than most fellows of the College and better than many.

Luke Cranwell of Loughborough Grammar School and Christ's College, Cambridge, was ejected from St Peter's church, Derby, by the Act of Uniformity, but, by all accounts, successfully practised medicine in the nearby little town of Kegworth until he died in 1683.[282] John Angell the younger, who probably obtained his MA at Magdalen Hall, Oxford, in 1625, became a schoolmaster at Leicester and keeper of the town library; then, after leaving the free school, became vicar of St Nicholas' church in 1638. Unlike his relative and namesake, he was not well thought of by his parishioners, and, by 1642, although still technically vicar, had turned to the profession of physician; a practice he continued in even when the easier time of the Restoration came.[283] Cranwell and Angell were men who were driven by necessity, but with Dr Clegg of Chapel-en-le-Frith, although he frankly admitted its value in supplementing his income, there were other forces at work too.

James Clegg (1679–1755) was educated from the age of fifteen to eighteen at the Reverend Richard Frankland's dissenting academy at Rathmell and was ordained in 1703 in Chapel-en-le-Frith. In a letter written to the Reverend Edmund Calamy in 1728, he explained at length why he had decided to take up the practice of physic. The idea seems to have been put into his head by Samuel Bagshaw of Ford, who thought many of the poor died for want of "a little seasonable help". In his diary, Clegg acknowledged the help Dr Adam Holland of Macclesfield had given him in his medical studies, and he certainly possessed Quincy's translation of Sanctorius's aphorisms, but, other than this, little is known of his training. Both Edinburgh and Glasgow refused him a degree, but in October 1729, to his great satisfaction, he was granted an MD by Aberdeen. Not only the poor received his ministrations but many families "of better note", such as the Bagshawes of The Oaks, Norton, and Joshua Wood of Bowden Hall. He travelled widely, visiting patients in Derby, Mansfield and Gainsborough, Knutsford and Macclesfield. His diary indicates that his treatment was simple for the day and on the whole successful, particularly in cases of smallpox. His surgical work was chiefly confined to dealing with fractures.[284]

These men, Ward, Cranwell, Angell, and Clegg were not, and never claimed to be apothecaries; they termed themselves physicians or doctors of physic. Their acquaintance with medical education varied from the best of the day, as in the case of Ward, to the mere gathering together of common-sense folk medicine, as with Clegg, but, because they had a degree, whether one in the Arts or one bought from Aberdeen, there is a tendency to give them a greater measure of respect than the "mere" shopkeeping apothecary.

[282] A. White, *History of the Loughborough Endowed Schools*, Loughborough Grammar School, 1969, p. 82.

[283] J. Simon, 'The two John Angels', *Trans. Leics. Arch. Hist. Soc.*, 1955, **31**: 45–46.

[284] V. S. Doe (editor), *The diary of James Clegg of Chapel-en-le-Frith, 1708–55*, Pt. 1, 1708–36, Matlock, Derbyshire Record Society, 1978, p. xliii. He was recommended for the degree by Dr Nettleton of Halifax, Dr Dixon of Bolton, and Dr Latham of Findern. Clegg had an assistant, Edward Bennett, who in later years described himself as a surgeon. He probably inherited Clegg's practice and was the ancestor of the Bennetts of Stodhart, medical men for over a century.

Beyond the fact that he learned his profession by apprenticeship, there is little information on the training of the provincial apothecary, though it is known that by the
mid-eighteenth century he not infrequently came to London for a short spell in order
to "walk the wards" or attend courses of lectures. Fortunately, the numerous letters
that passed between Richard Pulteney and his friends give quite a clear picture of how
a number of young men tried to fit themselves for their future career.

Richard Pulteney was born in Loughborough, Leicestershire, in 1730, the son of
Dissenters. He was educated at the local grammar school, which, like many another at
that period, was in a state of decline, probably in this case enhanced by the long
headship of Samuel Martin, who died in harness in 1749 aged seventy-four. Years
later, Pulteney wrote to "Sir" John Hill that, "The literary part of my education in
the early part of my life was greatly circumscribed".[285] Richard was a studious boy
with a great love of books but, even in the cities, in the eighteenth century, some titles
were in short supply; letters were full of requests to friends to try and buy them some
much-desired volumes. When obtained, they were lent round a circle of friends, and
the borrower, if he could find the time, would copy out those chapters that particularly
interested him. Richard, from the age of eleven, made abstracts from books on travel,
philology, and botany. His writing is clear and neat, and he obviously delighted in
reproducing maps.

There is no record of his binding to Mr Harris, an apothecary of Loughborough,
but it probably took place in 1745 or 1746. Nothing is known of Harris, whose son
Thomas, a cheerful, amusing, and intelligent young man, was a close friend of
Richard. One assumes Thomas received his initial training from his father, but by
1747, he was under the tutorship of an apothecary in Leicester. For five years, the two
apprentices wrote to each other frequently, exchanging views, experiences, and
textbooks.

On 21 July 1747, Thomas wrote a letter at "past 1 o'clock" and hardly able to keep
his eyes open, (because ". . . my man has took his pleasure today and I've weighed and
curs'd sugars") to tell Richard that he had found a copy of Mead's *De imperio* in
Unwin's shop. It was priced at the exorbitant sum of four shillings, so he suggested
that they should buy it between them, even though the bookseller admitted it was very
dear. The dealer was trying to be accommodating because he had told Harris that if
the book were not sold then he could have it all Sunday, whereupon Tom would send a
report of its contents to Pulteney by the newsman. Harris also tried to answer his
correspondent's query as to why a dog had not died when a mixture of nux vomica and
opium had been administered. The following year, they were both much concerned as
to the merits of vipers and their venom; references were made to Mead's views.
Thomas Harris had been noting the incidence of fits in infants. In his experience, the
babies were mostly affected at the full and change of the moon, and he wondered if,
". . . the Luminaries have any certain influences over the human body", but was
sceptical. A week later, writing on the same subject, he concluded that infant convul-
sions were due to too much water paps and lac humanum. He treated them with
adsorbents such as red coral, and laxatives of the syrup of violets or rhubarb type. He

---

[285] Linnean Society Library, Pulteney letters, copy of a letter to John Hill dated February 1758 sent by
Pulteney.

enquired of an old experienced apothecary what he thought was the reason for Mead's "Imperium Lunae", receiving the reply that it was but an old woman's tale. Harris was not entirely satisfied. He felt there must be ". . . some reason for such a change and sudden alteration in the human body", and wondered just what was the mechanism involved. He went on to add that the solution to the problem, ". . . must be the only way to perform the cure; if you know not this, how can you order any medicine, for it seems the most rational to me to consult with the disease before you cure".[286]

They discussed the merits of Florentine olive oil, some problem which Pulteney had encountered with Aethiops mineral, and the dangers of sophisticated gentian root. Gunthorpe, a local druggist, had sold some to two women," . . . they infused it in white wine and took a small dose which has almost killed 'em, though by the extraordinary care of an Apothecary they are perfectly recovered". John Fox, another Leicester apprentice, thought he had found some amongst his master's rad. gentian, and he and Harris intended to try it on the first dog they could obtain.[287] They liked to start their letters with a Latin tag or occasionally a Greek one, sometimes continuing in the former language. On December 1748, Thomas began with "Ophilobotanicos" and then told Richard he had decided to have his three volumes of Tournefort bound at a cost of thirteen shillings and would send one of them to Pulteney by Dicey's man. In return, he would like to have Dr Deering's treatise on smallpox. "Pray tell me why the small pox can be had but once, do you ever think that ever any one had 'em twice?" The questions of contagion and infection obviously interested Harris. In another letter, he was concerned to know, ". . . if the corrupted breath of a patient in a high fever taints the ambient air, so that when it comes to be inflated into the lungs causes the same disease in corpore sano . . . how does the poisonous air cause the same disease?"[288]

Richard was not always happy in his apprenticeship, but this he did not confide to Tom, but rather to another close friend, James Taylor, the nephew of Hugh Paull, apothecary of Kettering, and of a Mr Statham of Loughborough. Like Pulteney, but unlike Harris, Taylor was a Dissenter, and in 1747 was sent to the academy at Kibworth in south Leicestershire. The grammar schools being in disrepute and the English universities passing through one of their less luminous phases, the dissenting academies provided possibly the soundest education obtainable, if somewhat over-laden with religious instruction. James wrote that he planned to stay at Kibworth for a year, during which time he would study not only the classics but modern languages as well, including Italian. It was intended that he should have a career in medicine and he told Richard that he was to study, "Natural and Moral Philosophy which will not be intermixt with the Physical branch of any kind whatsoever, so that when I go to Edinburgh I shall have nothing to do but set about Physick entirely and make that with all its branches my sole study. I think this is very rational and I much approve of it not to mix Physick at an Academy with other studies." Through him, Pulteney was able to borrow a good variety of books.

[286] Letters from Harris to Pulteney, 2 July and 10 July, 1748.
[287] Harris to Pulteney, 15 October ?1749,
[288] Harris to Pulteney, 23 October ?1749.

The following year, Taylor went to Dr Philip Doddridge's famous academy at Northampton, and on 17 December, gave his friend a very detailed account of life there and the curriculum laid down for the full four years. This is of interest as it must have formed the basis of the general education received by many dissenting apothecaries, who, if they proceeded to a university, would travel to Scotland or Holland. In the junior class, the syllabus consisted of the classics, geography, shorthand, mathematics, logic, and oratory; the second year, they concerned themselves with ethics, evidences of Christianity, ecclesiastical history, Jewish antiquities, natural philosophy, and astronomy. The third year was similar to the second, except for the addition of algebra and metaphysics; the fourth was heavily orientated towards religious studies and was usually taken only by those who were to become ministers.[289]

Because of Pulteney's deep interest in botany, he had a correspondence with Dr George Deering, John Blackstone, John Hill, William Hudson, and, above all, William Watson. From these letters it can be seen that, though he had his own practice by the time he was twenty-two, his education was not regarded as finished. Watson gave the young apothecary much sage advice on how to extend his medical and chemical knowledge. He recommended that Pulteney should read Dr Lucas's *Essay on water* and Dr Home's work on bleaching, and told him that Dr Russell's treatise on the glands was a "must" for all medical practitioners.[290] Earlier, Pulteney had consulted Watson professionally on the use of electricity in medicine, having read in the *Gentleman's Magazine* of the removal of "ganglia" by "electrification".[291] Whether Richard had conducted experiments in electrostatics is not known, but Harris certainly had, for he had written on 15 June 1752, "I had the opportunity of trying some electrical experiments with one of my globes put in a clockmaker's lathe and gave myself such a shock as I would not repeat for all the world".

Pulteney had at least three apprentices, a Mr Godkin, Timothy Bentley, and Thomas Arnold. He seems to have had the happiest relations with them, and no doubt was as good an apprentice–master as lay in his power, but the last two must have regarded his shop and his surgical and medical practice as just a step towards their future education. Bentley, the son of a Leicester banker and mercer, in 1760, went to Warrington Academy and decided to proceed to Edinburgh in the following year. The year after that, he was joined by Thomas Arnold. Both wrote long letters to their late master, telling him of their professors and courses, with which they seem to have been well able to cope. Pulteney found these letters stimulating, and they undoubtedly contributed to his desire to extend his own interests. His situation in Leicester was far from comfortable. Pulteney's biographer, Dr Maton, thought this was because he was a Dissenter, but the letters from John Aiken, Pulteney's friend at the Kibworth and Warrington Academies, suggest that in some way he had transgressed medical etiquette. Aiken wrote in June 1760 that he was "much concerned at the continued uneasiness of your situation as I know rivalship with an old acquaintance and friend must be very grating to one of your mild and generous temper. . . ." Watson thought

---

[289] Taylor to Pulteney, 17 December 1748.
[290] Watson to Pulteney, 17 July 1756.
[291] Watson to Pulteney, 20 September 1755.

that the situation would never mend, but that Pulteney had insufficient money to buy an established apothecary's partnership in London. He preferred the suggestion of Dr George Baker of Stamford and Maxwell Garthshore of Uppingham, which Pulteney decided to follow. Watson wrote approvingly in February 1761, "I think very well of your intent to get a diploma from Scotland and afterwards to go to reside some little time at Leyden. The having been at a university, though but for a short time, will have its weight and if any difficulty should arise in procuring your diploma from Scotland you might take one regularly at Leyden as some friends of mine have done after a stay there not longer than six weeks."

Pulteney tarried long enough to be received into the Royal Society and write his thesis, and then, in March 1764, in the company of Garthshore, he went to Edinburgh, where the two men were well received by the professors. Pulteney was successful in his design, but not without some trouble:

> The opposition that was made to me was not I believe intended against me at first as I had passed my three private examinations before a word was said about it, until one Mr Hooper presented for trials, who had studied here but one year, this at length stirred up several others and I am sorry to say that I fear a little spice of envy might be at the bottom among three or four young gentlemen who have distinguished themselves in botany, and whom I had met too at Dr Hope's, the party were chiefly Americans; the most considerable Englishman I find was one who it seems is a neighbour of mine in a neighbouring county but I do not know him. However they have the most of them the generosity to allow and to express it in a paper which they delivered to the professors that I had a title to ask a degree but wished it to have been conferred in an honorary manner; the opposition sunk almost away before the graduation which was yesterday.[292]

He soon became an extra-licentiate of the College of Physicians, and then went to practise as a physician at Blandford Forum, Dorset. Beyond the fact that he had no longer an open shop and could certainly charge higher fees, one feels there was little difference in his practice. Undoubtedly, he relished his greater freedom – all botanist-apothecaries grumbled at the confinement of a shop, but it would not be true to say that his life for the first time became cultured. From his correspondence, it is clear that many apothecaries were men of culture. Their interests covered a broad spectrum; they wrote letters on subjects ranging from classical literature in the original Greek or Latin to religion, from botany to the influence of Lord Bute on the young king.

Thomas Harris, too, had literary interests. He told Pulteney in July 1750 that he had been reading Juvenal. "I must confess I have never read anything that afforded me so much pleasure in my life though I am forced to deny myself . . . . I have rose early and sat up late [so] that I find this month past it has surprisingly weakened my eyes. I cannot without great uneasiness read above half an hour by a candle. I should be glad to know if you think any kind of glasses would be of any service." Possibly Pulteney was interested in optics, as a couple of years earlier he had asked Thomas the value of a prism, to which the reply was, "A prism is worth five shillings I can't get a tube made yet, the Glass house is stop't working".[293]

Of Bentley, John Aiken wrote from Warrington Academy to Pulteney "I was (as

---

[292] Pulteney to Watson, 9 May 1764. It has been said that Richard Pulteney was the last man to receive a medical degree from Edinburgh University without putting in a period of study there, which was the point that had caused the disturbance.
[293] Harris to Pulteney, 7 September 1748.

you expected) agreeably surprised to Mr Bentley . . . . I am astonished at the improvement in the Greek which he reads with great readiness, as if he had studied it for some years under an able master. I less wonder at the progress he has made in botany, though it be really very great, as he had the advantage of your instruction".[294] In May 1761, Bentley told Richard that he had "not gone through a regular course of lectures and experiments in natural philosophy but have been acquainting myself with the theory". He was about to return to Leicester, and asked Pulteney to procure for him ". . . a Hippocrates and Galen in the original Greek with the Latin version in the best edition you can get".

Bentley's trip of three hundred miles to Edinburgh on horseback was full of interest for him. "York and Durham Cathedrals were the most entertaining sight I met with . . . which are very grand and magnificent. The very stones before the shrine in Durham cathedral are plainly hollowed by the scraping of the feet of those who bowed to St. Cuthbert, to whom the shrine was dedicated, and the innumerable minor saints that were placed around, as it were waiting on him."[295] In similar vein was the letter from James Taylor, when he made his first journey to Northampton. "Really to give you an impartial account of this famous borough, I think it exceeds Leicester in the uniformity of the Drapery and the Market Hill, and the church called All Hallows is in a far nobler taste than any I saw in Leicester. However Leicester will outvie Northampton in the stateliness and loftiness of houses, in the extent of the town, the riches of the inhabitants and the great trade it carries on with most of the principal towns of Great Britain."[296]

Pulteney was elected FRS in 1762, but he was by no means the first apothecary to be so honoured. A founder member was Nicasius Lefebvre, demonstrator of chemistry at the Jardin du Roi and later professor of chemistry to Charles II on his restoration;[297] and the second apothecary to be elected was John Haughton, in 1679. His particular interests were the improvement of husbandry and trade, for which he produced a weekly journal. He was followed by the four botanists, Samuel Doody (1695), James Petiver (1695), James Sherard (1709), and Isaac Rand (1719). Sylvanus Bevan (1725), John Martyn (1727), John Chandler (1735), and William Watson (1741) were also elected.

Of perhaps even greater interest is the Gentlemen's Society of Spalding. It was established in 1710, and so claims – it still exists – to be the oldest such society outside London and the universities. It called itself a "cell" of the Society of Antiquaries of London, of which most of its members were fellows. According to Gough and Nichols, it arose as a result of a few gentlemen of the town meeting in a coffee house to pass away an hour and read new publications. The founder, first president, and secretary for thirty-five years was Maurice Johnson of Spalding and the Inner Temple.[298] Meetings were held on Thursdays throughout the year, first at Younger's

---

[294] Aiken to Pulteney, 30 June 1760.
[295] Bentley to Pulteney, 4 December 1761.
[296] Taylor to Pulteney, [n.d.] summer 1748.
[297] Although not fellows of the Royal Society, the apothecaries of Oxford, John Crosse, Arthur Tillyard, and John Clerk, should be mentioned as they were so closely associated with the early members of Gresham College when it was exiled to Oxford.
[298] R. Gough and J. Nichols, 'The Gentlemen's Society at Spalding', in J. Nichols, *Literary anecdotes of*

coffee house in the abbey yard, and then in a private house. In the 1740s, they took over part of the old monastery and fitted it up with a library and a museum. In 1750, it is related that the meetings began about four o'clock and lasted until ten. The "Oeconomical Rules" still exist and show how the society was conducted. Each meeting began with drinking a dish of tea or coffee; later in the evening, "a tankard of ale holding one quart, and no more, must be set upon the tables". Twelve clean pipes and an ounce of tobacco and a chamber-pot were also to be provided, as well as a Latin dictionary and a Greek lexicon.[299]

The society did not confine itself to antiquities, "... but made discoveries in Natural History and improvements in Arts and Sciences in general ... they only excluded politics".[300] Nichols added that the apothecaries had a physic garden in Spalding in 1745, and that the society had a fine hortus siccus. On admission, members gave a valuable book and paid a shilling per meeting and twelve shillings a year subscription. A list is given for members, both regular and honorary, for the years 1710–53; it included such famous names as Isaac Newton, Hans Sloane, John Evelyn, George Vertue the engraver, the two Wesleys, and a Mr Rand, who may have been the director of the Chelsea Physic Garden. In 1729, Johnson told a friend that they had recently admitted two doctors of divinity, one of them "head" of Queen's College, Oxford, two seamen, a lawyer, a captain, two surgeons, and five other gentlemen, whereby they were enabled to carry on a correspondence in most parts of the world. The number of members who practised medicine is noticeable, not least among them apothecaries and surgeons. The physicians included Panagioti Condoiti, physician to the Empress of Russia, and men from the eastern counties such as Charles Balguy MD of Peterborough; Dixon Coleby MD, John King MD, Thomas Wallis MD, all of Stamford; and the Reverend Charles Townshend, curate of Spalding and Deeping, MB of Emmanuel College, Cambridge. The surgeons included Claudius Amyand, serjeant-surgeon to the king, Francis Drake of York, author of a history of that city, Robert Guy of St Bartholomew's Hospital, and local men such as John Hepburn of Stamford and Harry Bayley of Spalding. The "operator" at the society was for many years a surgeon, Michael Cox.

Men specifically named as apothecaries were fewer, but included Peter Bold, James Brecknock of Holbeach, Heneage Browne, Isaac Heath, "Sir" John Hill, Calamy Ives of Wisbech, John Rogerson, and John Ward of Spalding. There were two druggists, Edward Pincke and Anselm Beaumont,[301] but no other shopkeepers.

Further information on the apothecaries' cultural background can be gathered from the book subscription project currently in progress at the University of Newcastle

the eighteenth century, London, J. Nichols, 1812, vol. 6, pp. 1–162, list of members pp. 69–122. In 1712, there were twelve regular members and eighteen extra-regular members; subsequently there was a "running" list of 355.

[299] R. E. Duthie, 'English florists' societies and feasts ...', *Garden History*, 1982, **10**: 34.

[300] Dr Middleton Massey gave a rather different picture when he wrote to James Petiver, "... as for subscribing to yr. British plants my circumstances will not give me leave and the gentlemen of the Club are not at all curious in natural history ...." (British Library, Sloane MSS., MS. 4067, f. 48.)

[301] Edward Pincke formed a trading partnership with his master Anthony Kingsley, wholesale druggist, and a journeyman Anselm Beaumont in 1716. See Matthews, op. cit., note 154 above, p. 215. In August 1730, Anselm, son of Anselm Beaumont of London, was apprenticed to Thomas Graham, citizen and apothecary.

upon Tyne. A preliminary guide to apothecaries in the book subscription lists was produced for the Cambridge conference of the British Society for the History of Pharmacy in 1974. It is by no means complete, as names had been extracted from only some ninety lists out of nearly five thousand known, nor had it been edited. Names were only given if there were a designation such as chemist, druggist, surgeon or surgeon and apothecary, or apothecary. The last was by far the most frequent. Between the years 1709 and 1748, there were apothecaries and surgeon-apothecaries in England and Wales who subscribed to seventy-five different publications. They ranged from James Durham's *Christ crucify'd* to Pemberton's *An essay for the further improvement of dancing,* from John Strype's *A survey of . . . London and Westminster* to Peter Barwick's *Vita Johannis Barwick.* Religion was not overwhelmingly popular, though John Sturt's *The book of common prayer,* George Smalridge's *Sixty sermons . . .,* and John Walker's *. . . Sufferings of the clergy* were all represented. Natural history had its following, for example Eleazor Albin's *Natural history of spiders* and his work on English insects, but it is obvious that history had by far the greatest number of adherents. Thomas Hearne's books were well patronized, whilst others included Simon Ockley's *History of the Saracens, The history of the royal genealogy of Spain* by Thomas Richers, and Bulstrode Whitelocke's *Memorials of the English affairs . . . of King Charles.* Silvanus Bevan, Rice Charlton of Bristol, and John Wilmer all subscribed to *A view of Sir Isaac Newton's philosophy* by Henry Pemberton, and John Markham of Paternoster Row was such a bookworm that he subscribed to no less than twenty-one books between 1716 and 1728.[302]

The view of a contemporary can perhaps give us our most valuable assessment of the education of an apothecary both before and after he started to practise. In 1682, Hugh Squier wrote, "In my Study at Westminster on St. Stephen's Day. Resolved: That there shall be a school house built in South Molton Church Yard (if there be not found a more convenient Place for it in the town) of stonework all most strong as a little chapel . . . to contain 150 boys. . . . And this shall be no horn book school to teach little children to read nor shall any one be admitted but such as can read in the psalter, . . . nor shall it be to teach persons the Latin tongue or the rules of Grammar, but this school shall be chiefly to teach good writing and Arithmetick . . . Arithmetick is as necessary as our daily bread, or salt unto our meat, the thing every man is making use of every hour of all his life . . . ." To Squier, it was the saddest thing "To see the godly good old wife (in the middest of all her pressing affairs) take pains to pack her boys away to school . . . there to learn, not to read divinity nor so much as history nor the tale of Tom Thumb, which would prove far more profitable than some Horum, harum, horum, genetivo, hujus huick etc., when it is sure they can maintain them but two years at the school in all . . . I say either go on and perfect Grammar with the Latin tongue, or else 'tis madness to begin, for unless a man means to be a divine, or a lawyer or an apothecary or a gentleman he makes no use thereof, but forgets again all that he learnt."[303]

---

[302] Wellcome Institute Library, interim print-out of the project.

[303] J. Cock, *Records of ye antient borough of South Molton in ye county of Devon,* South Molton, for the author, 1893, pp. 176–179.

VI

STATUS AND SOCIAL POSITION

The standard opinion concerning the apothecary's status is embodied in the statement by Hamilton that in 1660, "... a physician was a gentleman, while apothecaries and surgeons were mere craftsmen", with its further elaboration: that "At that time [1617] they [the apothecaries] were compounders and dispensers of medicine, and the stigma of 'tradesmen' clung to them long after the sale of drugs had ceased to be the main function of the individual apothecary, though not of the company". She then said that after the Civil War the status of the apothecary was rising, but "The apothecaries seem to have been mainly sons of small shopkeepers, yeomen and respectable craftsmen. In towns the practising apothecary was of low status: but in the country, where he was usually the only doctor, he was sometimes a man of good family who had qualified in the cheapest and most useful way; there he might take his position according to his family rather than according to his occupation. But the average apothecary did not come of a good or wealthy family; indeed the profession was one way for the lowest classes to climb".[304] The physicians of the College would have readily concurred with this view. As Cameron has written, "The Physicians decried the Apothecaries as men ignorant, unlettered, and unlearned in the science of medicine and in opprobrium called them empirics".[305]

The jealous, ill-founded diatribes of the nervous fellows of the College have echoed and re-echoed down through the centuries and can be heard to this day. "Just as a tinker-soldier or a sailor-ploughboy is impossible, so a gentleman-apothecary is unthinkable." "Edmund Withering [an apothecary], who for his station and time was wealthy met and even more unusually married Miss Hector, the sister of Dr Brooke Hector of Lichfield."[306] "At this time [1768] ... the apothecaries of the era were not recognised as professional men, and, in an age of quacks, they were barely respectable."[307] "George Cooke of Fitton, the object of Corbett's frequent gibes because he had been an apothecary, made his submission and was restored to his living."[308]

The denigration of the apothecaries continued with a group who were in some degree, their successors, the chemists and druggists. W. J. Reader, in his study of the rise of the professional classes in nineteenth-century England, when considering the effects of the Medical Act of 1886, wrote that it, "... finally shut out the chemists and druggists from the medical profession", and that "... their separation from the doctors, though undesired, was not undignified, but in the nature of things they could never escape the taint of retail trade."[309] There is little doubt that the common view is

---

[304] B. Hamilton, 'The medical professions in the eighteenth century', *Econ. Hist. Rev.*, 1951, **4**: 141–169, see pp. 141, 158, 159.

[305] Wall, Cameron, and Underwood, op. cit., note 8 above, vol. 1, p. 4.

[306] T. W. Peck and K. Wilkinson, *William Withering of Birmingham*, Bristol, J. Wright, 1950, pp. 31, 33.

[307] P. Lewis, 'An Aldeburgh apothecary', *Hist. Med.*, 1971, **3**: 23.

[308] R. W. Ketton-Cremer, *Norfolk and the Civil War*, London, Faber, 1969, p. 81.

[309] W. J. Reader, *Professional men. The rise of the professional classes in nineteenth century England*, London, Weidenfeld & Nicolson, 1966, p. 68.

held that there is a lowering of social status by standing behind the counter of a shop – and that it has always been so. The conclusions to be drawn from this belief are that these shopkeepers, whether apothecary or pharmacist, must have come from near the bottom rungs of society, that they were ignorant and probably quite unethical, even unscrupulous in their efforts to amass money, because they had no professional standards, nor did they associate with those who had.

It has often been claimed that England had in the past (and some say still has) a class-ridden society with inflexible barriers erected between the strata. In fact, this picture is far from the truth. Charles Wilson has written,

> The society [of the period 1603–1763] was roughly stratified by contemporaries into the nobility, gentry, merchants, professions, yeomen, freeholders, customary tenants, leaseholders, shopkeepers, craftsmen, labourers and that great mass – perhaps a third or more of the total – they called 'the poor'. Yet nobles apart, these labels did not imply legal definition of social status, though a man might be labelled knight, esquire, gentleman, yeoman or husbandman, in order to be assessed when a direct tax was being raised. Throughout the period there was a remarkable degree of social mobility, especially between the middle and top ranges of society. Many families contained representatives of the peerage, gentry, merchants, and professions, to say nothing of poor relations, at the same moment in time. . . . The social categories invented by nineteenth century historians – feudal, bourgeois, working class – do not sit happily on such a society. The simple idea of large and more or less solid social 'classes' distinguished from each other by different interests is not only unhelpful in interpreting the course of events: it can be positively misleading.[310]

In England, there was no definition of a "gentleman", any more than there was of a "yeoman", but for convenience this has been attempted by Anthony Wagner, Garter King-of-Arms. The inheritor of a knight's fee, or manor, had never been automatically a knight, but was usually knighted by his father or his lord after training, first as a valet and then as an esquire. As time elapsed, the financial burdens of knighthood could weigh so heavily that many did not take it up when they came of age, thus the apprentice to knighthood, an esquire, came to mean a man of knightly rank but one who did not intend to become one. Some time after 1400, the need arose for a general term for a class which centred on the esquires and others who ranked with them, for this the designation "gentleman" or "gentry" came to be used. The valet or yeoman was ranked immediately below the esquire and was regarded as the knight's servant or retainer. In Tudor times, the name was applied to the class of country freeholders who came next in rank to the gentry. Rich yeomen were frequently richer than poor gentry, and intermarriage was not uncommon.[311]

An Act of Parliament and a book of etiquette of the fifteenth century put the merchants, who were in effect the ruling class of the towns, on a level with the esquires. Some, such as London aldermen, could stand higher, and a few of great wealth and power ranked with the upper nobility. As Trevelyan has said, "Yeomen, merchants and lawyers who had made their fortunes, were perpetually recruiting the ranks of the landed gentry; while the younger sons of the manor house were apprenticed into industry and trade."[312] It is important to note that, to quote Wilson again, "Trade did not derogate from that status [of gentry]. A Cheshire gentleman could describe himself in 1640 as a gentleman by birth and a linen draper by trade. In

[310] Wilson, op. cit., note 58 above, preface, p. xiv.
[311] A. Wagner, *English ancestry*, Oxford University Press, 1961, pp. 46–48, 58–59.
[312] G. M. Trevelyan, *English social history*, London, Reprint Society, 1948, p. 165.

a case in 1634 a witness said that 'many citizens of great worth and esteem descended of very ancient gentle families, being soap boilers by trade even and yet accounted gentlemen'."[313]

In France, nobility was sharply defined and possessed important legal and fiscal privileges, thus the importance of coats-of-arms as labels gradually lapsed. In England, the opposite happened; as there was no legal definition of gentility, then the outward marks became more important, of which Defoe wrote so pungently, "We see the tradesmen of England as they grow wealthy coming every day to the Heralds' Office, to search for the Coats of Arms of their ancestors, in order to paint them upon their coaches, and engrave them upon their plate, . . . or carve them upon the pediments of their new houses; and how often do we see them trace the registers of their families up to the prime nobility, or the most antient gentry of the Kingdom."[314] Henry VII, in 1492, had declared that a grant of arms by Garter King-of-Arms established the grantee's gentility beyond question. Heraldic visitations had been already established but now the kings-of-arms were given powers of inquisition to determine whether the bearer was entitled to them, either by ancestral right or by the grant of someone of sufficient authority. After 1530, Clarenceux King-of-Arms in a visitation had to deface or remove any arms that were false or devised without authority. Thereafter, until 1686, visitations were made about once every generation, when arms and pedigrees were examined; if found to be valid they were entered in the visitation books, if false, then the usurper had to make a disclaimer. Apothecaries or their antecedents, men such as Richard Meynell, John Ne[e]dham, Richard and John Conyers, are to be frequently found in the visitation books. By the eighteenth century, the whole system of surveillance had broken down, which inevitably led to false claims and bitter acrimony.

In 1795, John Mason Good, in his book *History of medicine in so far as it relates to the profession of the apothecary*, claimed that apothecaries' profits were no longer attracting sons of respectable families, so making it impossible for apothecaries to demand high premiums for apprenticeships. The validity of this statement is arguable, for a study of the Inland Revenue apprenticeship records for the eighteenth century shows that sizeable sums of consideration money were obtained. As a general rule, it can be said that the larger the sum paid, the higher the social position of the apprentice-master and of his craft or trade.

In mid-century, the apothecary's average premium lay between £50 and £105, the provinces being, in general, rather lower than London, and may be usefully compared with other professions, crafts, and trades. Weavers, nailers, and framework-knitters were amongst the lowest, being a mere £3–4, and even as little as £1 10s. Joiners, butchers, and watchmakers could rise to £16 or £20 but were more usually half those sums; grocers varied from £10 to £50, and saddlers and coachmakers from £25 to £50. Merchants had a wide variation, £40 to £260, with the premiums of the overseas trading organizations, such as the Merchant Adventurers, running to £500 and £600. Attorneys were, on the whole, consistently between £100 and £150. The surgeons of the great London hospitals could command figures between £250 and £400, but the

---

[313] Wilson, op. cit., note 58 above, p. 14.
[314] Ibid., p. 15.

APPRENTICESHIP PREMIUMS FROM THE INLAND REVENUE RECORDS IN THE EARLY EIGHTEENTH AND EARLY NINETEENTH CENTURIES[315]

Volume I. October 1711–November 1712 (London)			*Volume 41.* May 1710–January 1712 (Provinces)	
Premiums	Apothecaries	Surgns & Apoths.	Apothecaries	Surgns & Apoths.
£40–£50	14	–	20	–
£50–£75	26	2	19	2
	40	2	39	2
	Out of a total of 58 premiums in which the minimum is £20 and the maximum £100	Out of a total of 2 minimum £50 maximum £65	Out of a total of 57 minimum £20 maximum £65	Out of a total of 4 minimum £27 10s. maximum £60

Volume 38. March 1799–April 1802 (London)			*Volume 71.* May 1803–September 1805 (Provinces)	
Premiums	Apothecaries	Surgns & Apoths.	Apothecaries	Surgns & Apoths.
£50–£100	6	24	1	27
£100–£150	12	33	4	44
£150–£200	4	11	–	23
£200–£250	3	17	–	12
	25	85	5	106
	Out of a total of 35 in which the minimum is £50 and the maximum £400	Out of a total of 110 minimum £10 maximum £250	Out of a total of 6 minimum £25 maximum £105	Out of a total of 176 minimum £15 maximum £367 10s

ordinary rank and file were nearer £30 and £50.

For the first thirty years that the Inland Revenue records were kept, the trade, profession, or status of the apprentice's father was usually stated, a practice which unfortunately later died out. Jenkinson, in his examination of the Surrey apprenticeship records between 1710 and 1740, noted that the sons of gentlemen were in four cases apprenticed (or articled) to attorneys, which is not unexpected, whilst three were bound to goldsmiths, four to apothecaries, three to barber-surgeons, and five to mariners.[316] Members of three of the London livery companies, the merchant-tailors, drapers, and haberdashers, had three gentlemen's sons apiece, and the stationers, four. Clerks, that is clergymen, placed their sons in much the same occupations as gentlemen. Besides mercers, woollen- and linen-drapers, the lesser merchants, carpenters, tallow-chandlers, and ironmongers, all of whom could attract reasonably substantial premiums, gentlemen could place their offspring with tanners, blacksmiths, butchers, gardeners, and curriers, and even such lowly beings as cordwainers and framework-knitters. Nevertheless, these were the exceptions. An analysis of the parentage of apothecarial apprentices in the first three years of the Inland Revenue

[315] Volumes 1 to 40 of the Inland Revenue apprenticeship records are termed "London volumes", and numbers 41 to 72 "provincial"; in the first case the tax was brought direct to the London office, and in the second was taken to a local collecting centre. In fact, particularly as the eighteenth century progressed, the geography of the place of apprenticeship is very mixed.

[316] C. H. Jenkinson (editor), *Surrey apprenticeships*, Surrey Record Society, 1929, vol. 10, *passim*. By "mariner" was meant the captain of a merchant ship.

records gives further details of the background from which they were drawn.[317] The parental position of the 223 apprentices may be divided in the following manner:

52 belonged to the professions (apothecaries, attorneys, clergy, doctors of physic, master mariners, scriveners, and surgeons, and two citizen and barber-surgeons which are doubtful).[318]

31 were craftsmen (brewer, blacksmith, chainmaker, clothworker, coachmaker, cordwainer, farrier, glazier, glover, girdler, herald-painter, joiner, pin-maker, sergemaker, shearmaker, shipwright, stationer, tanner, tailor, thread-twister, wire-drawer).[319]

22 were shopkeepers (baker, butcher, draper, grocer, haberdasher, innholder, leatherseller, mercer, victualler, vintner, woollen-draper).[320]

13 were merchants (drugster, goldsmith, grazier, maltster, merchant, and merchant taylor, to which should be added two aldermen of London who were almost certainly in this class).[321]

43 were described as gentlemen, to which may be added two esquires.[322]

12 were termed yeoman.

46 no description given, this figure includes seven widows.

As can be readily appreciated, considerable difficulty was experienced in drawing up the above categories and they are by no means rigid, but, taken at their face value, it can be seen that out of a total of 187 known occupations and positions of status, the apprentices' parents totalled 112 in the professional/merchant/gentleman class, and sixty-six in that of the craftsman/shopkeeper/yeoman.

Holmes has noted the very close link between the sons of the parsonage and the apothecaries' practices: ". . . in fact in the latter years of Anne, the clergy supplied apothecaries countrywide with more apprentices than did any other occupational group".[323] He added that "Non-armigerous country gentlemen . . . now readily placed their boys with good City apothecaries", and agreed largely with the 1724 claim of the Society of Apothecaries that their membership ". . . chiefly consists of those that have been the son of the reverend the clergy, and of gentlemen". Holmes believed that the status of the apothecary had so greatly improved in the fifty years between 1680 and 1730 that ". . . forty years before [1724] the claim would not have been made at all". This belief is not substantiated by the bindings of the London Apothecaries' Society, as a great many gentlemen's sons, most of them armigerous, may be noted in the records, for example, Richard Meynell (1648), Richard Squire (1657), Thomas Denman (1657), Benjamin Charlewood (1672), and Charles Nedham (1679) in the years prior to 1680.[324]

Gentlefolk of the period under review did not regard apprenticeship as demeaning.

[317] Vols. 41 and 42 = May 1710 to June 1713; vols. 1 and 2 = October 1711 to May 1714.

[318] No less than thirty-two clergy placed their sons with apothecaries.

[319] Many of these craftsmen, if not most of them, would be well-to-do masters. Those described as belonging to a London company are taken at their face value.

[320] Some of these shopkeepers could have been listed as craftsmen, e.g. bakers. The stationers were also a borderline case, they could be either printers or publishers.

[321] The citizen and merchant-taylor may have had nothing to do with the clothing industry, in 1710 out of a livery of 485, 300 members were not tailors. See F. Simpson, *Chester city gilds: the Barber-Surgeons' Company*, Chester, G. R. Griffith, 1911, p. 5.

[322] The lack of precision in the use of the term "gentleman" can be seen in the case of Charles Croughton. In the Inland Revenue records, when he was apprenticed to Ralph Sudlow in 1712, he was stated to be the son of Charles Croughton, gentleman, but when he gained the freedom of Chester on 1 March 1722, he was recorded as "Charles Croughton of Chester, apothecary, son of Charles Croughton of Chester, silkweaver".

[323] Holmes, op. cit., note 2 above, p. 212.

[324] For further details, see J. G. L. Burnby, 'Three 17th century London apothecaries', *Pharm. Hist.*, 1975, **5**: pt. 1, pp. 2–3.

The signing of articles for training or of indentures for apprenticeship does not seem to have been regarded as significantly different. The Inland Revenue books show that in the eighteenth century, articles were in the main used by merchants and attorneys, and on occasion by surgeons, but that they were not confined to the future professions; bricklayers, butchers, dyers, and joiners could also use them, if less frequently.[325] Many families of impeccable status thought apprenticeship a fine method of entering a career, as witness the Frewens.

Thomas Frewen (1704–91), who has been mentioned in connexion with smallpox inoculation (p. 75), practised as an apothecary and surgeon until at least 1755, when he gained an MD from Leiden. He was apprenticed to George Lake senior of Sevenoaks, surgeon, for seven years in 1719, and his brother Edward was bound to John Spencer, citizen and barber-surgeon six years later.[326] Little is known of Edward's career but the *Medical Register* of 1779 shows him to be at Lewes (probably in partnership with Thomas, who had been forced to move from Rye to Lewes), that he was a member of the London Surgeons' Company, and that he too had obtained an MD. The two brothers were the sons of Thankfull Frewen (1669–1749) of Northiam, Sussex, clerk. Thankfull's father, Thomas (1630–77), grandfather, John (1595–1654), and great-grandfather, John (1560–1628) had all been rectors of Northiam. Thankfull's unusual Christian name was that of his great uncle (1591–1656), purse-bearer and secretary to Lord-Keeper Thomas Coventry, and brother to Accepted (1583–1664), Archbishop of York. As might be guessed, John, the father of Accepted and Thankfull, had been an extreme Puritan and for a period was in danger of losing his living.[327] The Frewen family, so eminently professional, middle class and, latterly, conforming, who could afford university education if so desired, nevertheless chose apprenticeship for two of its sons.

As has been already noted (p. 17), both Roberts and Rook have found in the Tudor and Stuart periods that the background of physicians and apothecaries was remarkably similar, that they were often close friends and frequently helped each other with the administrative and legalistic problems of life and death. Older historians would have found this an unexpected conclusion. In 1950, Poynter and Bishop wrote a paper on John Symcotts (1592?–1662) MD (Cantab.) of Huntingdon. They considered in some detail the training of a physician at Oxford and Cambridge, and they appear to have found the Symcotts family history consonant with that of a physician.

John's twin brother Robert was also admitted to Queens' College in 1608, was ordained priest in 1614, and was rector of Sandy from 1628 till his death eleven years later. Robert's only son William succeeded to most of John's by no means inconsiderable estate; he had been to Trinity College and was an MA by 1659; although Poynter believed him to be the possessor of an MD, no proof has been found. One of John's

---

[325] Jenkinson (op. cit., note 316 above) has written that it is difficult to define the exact difference between indentures and articles at this period, as the latter were not defined in the law dictionaries of the eighteenth century. He inclined to the view that articles were used when the conventional phraseology of indentures did not cover a particular need.

[326] PRO, Inland Revenue apprenticeship records, I.R./1/7, f. 62, premium £73 10*s*. Thomas Frewen is known to have taken at least two apprentices himself, Samuel Munn in 1743 and Charles Hill in 1748; I.R./1/10, f. 110, premium £105.

[327] *DNB*, vol. 20, pp. 272–275; *Burke's landed gentry*, 4th ed., 1863, p. 518.

brothers, George, was a "London merchant", and another, Thomas, was a "London wine-merchant".

Further investigation has shown that Thomas, probably the oldest of the family, was a citizen and vintner, and at the time of his death in 1658, was a governor of St Bartholomew's Hospital. George was a citizen and merchant-taylor, and from his will of 1657, a wealthy man. Although a member of the Merchant-Taylors' Company, he may well have been a vintner too, for he left the lease of his tavern, the Three Tunns in Newgate Market, to his brother Thomas, who was already living there. George's daughter Mary received £800, his son Thomas £450 (". . . and he knows why I give him no more."), son John the lease of the Windmill, Fleet Street, and ". . . any debts he owes me". His eldest son, another George, educated at Eton, had died soon after gaining an MA at King's College, Cambridge, in 1655, leaving a wife and child, but the most interesting to us of the older George's four sons, is Robert.

On 9 October 1655, Robert was bound apprentice to William Rowsewell, citizen and apothecary, for eight years.[328] He took up his freedom of the Society in 1663 and was an active member, carrying out such duties as being steward on the Lord Mayor's day in 1673 and for the herborizing at Greenwich in 1679. Robert was bequeathed by his father in 1657, £300 when he was twenty-one for the setting up of a shop, a venture which must have been made much easier by the receipt of a £24 annuity from the will of his uncle John, the physician.[329] No doubt Poynter would have found Robert the apothecary's position in this family as surprising as he found that of Gideon Delaune, when he wrote,

> His younger brothers Isaac and Peter . . . were trained to professions, Isaac to medicine [MD, Leiden] and Peter to the Church. Another brother, Paul, . . . was also trained to medicine and became an MD of Padua and Cambridge and a Fellow of the College of Physicians. We are left to speculate how it was that Gideon, the eldest son and heir, was not given an equally good start in a career. We shall see that he was respected and trusted by his father and there was no question of lack of means. He was later to do better, financially, than any of his family . . . .[330]

Genealogy has long been besmirched with the cry of "antiquarianism", but the revived enthusiasm for family history, as it now prefers to be known, is beginning to fight back. Elizabeth Simpson has made the plea that the family historian has a role to play that is valuable to all the other groups of historians, local, social, medical, industrial, demographical, and so on, and that ultimately there should be a total acceptance of family history as just one more branch of history.[331] Since the social scene in England shows such fluidity, it is essential, in order to determine more exactly the social niche occupied by the apothecary, that family case histories be made. Only

[328] F. N. L. Poynter and W. J. Bishop, 'A 17th century doctor and his patients: John Symcotts, 1592?–1662', *Beds. Hist. Rec. Soc. Pubns.*, 1951, **31**: introduction, pp. x–xvi.; Guildhall Library, Society of Apothecaries' court minutes, MS. 8200/2, f. 29. He asked permission of the court on 8 August 1671 to take a second apprentice. He was one of the many apothecaries who stayed in London throughout the Great Plague.

[329] PRO, PCC, Prob. 11 269, f. 452, will of George Symcotts, proved 3 March 1658; PCC, Prob. 11 309, f. 159, will of John Symcotts, doctor of physic, proved 15 December 1662. Besides the annuity, Robert received from his uncle ". . . thirty four shilling pieces of King James and eight old angels, one is a double duckett to keep for my sake".

[330] F. N. L. Poynter, *Gideon Delaune and his family circle*, London, Wellcome Historical Medical Library, 1965, p. 10.

[331] E. Simpson, 'Family history societies', *Local Historian*, 1981, **14**: 261.

when we know something of a man's background, relatives, friends, interests, and civic affairs can a reasonable assessment be made, and the old, glib, inaccurate generalities be discarded.

For our first case history we will take the London apothecary, John Conyers, a man, as far as his Society was concerned, of the middle rank but who was on the fringe of the exciting scientific world of his day. Conyers wrote in his memoranda on 25 January 1677, "... my Father 45 years since, Mr Edward Conyers or Coniers, was espoused to Mrs Jane Clarke my mother" at the church of St Faith's, which then lay under the ruins of St Paul's Cathedral. The following day, he made a reference to his two brothers, "Meeting with my Brother Mr Emanuel Conyers the Confectioner hee ... tould mee my Brother Conyers at the Tower, the storekeeper, both of them was at Epping forest hunting of the haire. . . .".[332]

Of the father little is known, but all three of his sons were members of London companies, Edward was made free of the Leathersellers' in 1667, Emanuel of the Grocers' in 1664, and John of the Apothecaries' in 1658. Although their parents were married in London, it is known that they were living in Leicestershire at the time of the boys' bindings.[333] This is not surprising, because a pedigree of John Nichols shows that the elder Edward Conyers was the descendant of an armigerous family of Wakerley, Northamptonshire, near the county border.[334]

John Conyers' first shop was at the sign of the Unicorn in Fleet Street, from which he practised all through the Great Plague. He is known to have issued a pamphlet entitled *Direction for the prevention and cure of the plague, fitted for the poorer sort*, which is an indication of the standing of his customers. It is probable that his shop was swept away by the Great Fire, for we next hear of him at the sign of the White Lion in the same street. Early in 1666, he married Mary Glisson, the niece of Francis Glisson, Regius Professor of Physick at Cambridge, who later lived nearby in Newe Street.[335] Another neighbour was Thomas Tompion, the clockmaker, to whom he lent one of his hygroscopes, and not much farther away, that controversial figure, William Salmon. Salmon was a prolific author, and in the preface of his *The practice of curing diseases* (1681) he complained ". . . of a late scandalous Abuse put upon Me by one Con . . . s a Potecary or Pot-carryer of Fleet St. who reports . . . that only as an Amanuensis I wrote them by the Instruction of another Gentleman. . . ." From which it seems that Conyers approved of Salmon's books but found the man's flamboyancy

---

[332] British Library, Sloane MSS., Conyers' memoranda, MS. 958, ff. 127, 127v.

[333] Communication from the clerk to the Leathersellers' Company; Guildhall Library, the Grocers' Company records, bindings, MS. 11593/1, f. 262 (2); Apothecaries' Society court minutes, MS. 8200/1, f. 477r, "2 August 1649, John Conyers, son of Edward Conyers of Little Bowden in the county of Northampton, exam'd . . . bound to Robert Phelps for 8 years from 29 September 1649". Little Bowden is now in Leicestershire; later Edward senior was living at Elmthorpe.

[334] Nichols, op. cit., note 91 above, vol. 2, p. 456. The Conyers brothers were descended from Reginald of Wakerley, who died in 1514, see pedigree.

[335] Francis Glisson was one of nine sons and four daughters, the children of William Glisson of Rampisham, Dorset (J. P. Rylands (editor), *Visitation of Dorset, 1623*, London, Harleian Society Publications, 1885, vol. 20, p. 46). Two of Francis' brothers, Paul and John, were in the church. Francis, and probably John Conyers too, was a Parliamentarian; he was a classical fellow of Caius College, Cambridge, and did not obtain his MD until 1634, when he was thirty-seven. He probably spent little time in Cambridge after 1640; he was president of the College of Physicians and a founder fellow of the Royal Society.

THE CONYERS OF WAKERLEY, BLASTON, AND LONDON

REGINALD CONYERS of Wakerley, N'hants.

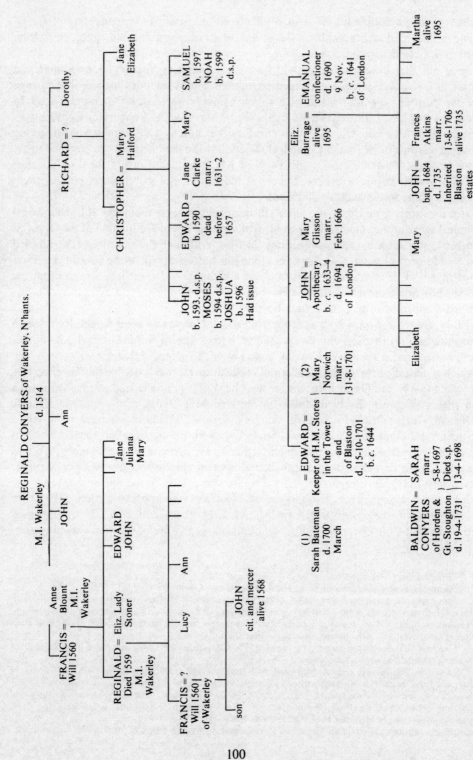

The earlier part of the pedigree is based on that in Nichols, op. cit., footnote 91, p. 456. Later part amended to accord with more recent research.

so disagreeable that he did not wish to believe that Salmon had written them.[336]

John Conyers' brother, Edward, the Keeper of His Majesty's stores in the Tower, made money and became determined to return to the root-stock of their family by becoming a landed gentleman. In the 1680s, he bought the manors of Blaston and Bradley in south Leicestershire. Unfortunately for his aspirations of re-founding a county dynasty, he had but one child, Sarah. Nothing daunted, a marriage was arranged between her and a certain Baldwin Conyers, who was in no way related.[337] Tragically, the centre of all Edward's plans died in 1698, only eight months after her marriage, to be followed by Edward's wife a year later. Edward married for the second time in August 1701, but only lived a further six weeks.[338]

Both of Edward Conyers' brothers predeceased him, John, our apothecary, in 1694, and Emanuel, the confectioner in All Hallows Staining, in 1690. Although John had had a large family, only two daughters lived to adulthood, and consequently Edward's considerable estate passed to a son of Emanuel, also named John, who was born in 1684.[339] Although this younger John married in 1706, there was again a failure in the male line, and by the strange terms of Edward's will, the Leicestershire estate passed to yet another Conyers family. Once again, there was no relationship, but the Conyers of Walthamstow were well known, for they were immensely wealthy.[340]

Such was the family of apothecary John Conyers, one which sprang from good county stock, made a fair competence in the great city, but in the long term failed to re-establish a dynasty of landowners. (For Conyers' scientific work, see pp. 44–46.)

Holmes has noted that the sector of society that comprised both "bona-fide professionals and pseudo-professionals" expanded more rapidly in numbers, wealth, and relative weight in the late seventeenth and first half of the eighteenth centuries than any other. He remarked also that by 1730, owing to the growth of urbanization, there was offered more opportunity for social intercourse between the practitioners of law, religion, and medicine, which slowly led to an awareness of the separate social identity of professional people.[341] Interchange and cross-fertilization of beliefs and standards occurred between clergy and attorneys, medical practitioners of all hues, and the parsonage or manse, all of which was enriched by the newly emergent engineers, schoolmasters, civil servants, and officers of the army and navy. Although

---

[336] W. Kirkby, 'A quack of the 17th century', *Pharm. J.*, 1910, **84**: 259. Although over-fond of self-advertisement, Salmon was no illiterate mountebank. His *Botanologia* shows him to have been to the Carolinas, and he is likely to have been originally a ship's surgeon, a suggestion supported by his will, in which he bequeathed £1,000 obtained from the sale of his library to his brother Francis Salmon of Gosport, physician (PRO, PCC., Prob. 11 532 f. 91).

[337] Baldwin Conyers' father was John Conyers of Gray's Inn, son of Christopher of Horden, Durham.

[338] His first wife, Sarah, had been the daughter of a fellow citizen and leather-seller, Matthew Bateman; the second, Madam Mary Norwich, sister of Sir Erasmus Norwich of Brampton, Northamptonshire, baronet.

[339] Nichols (loc. cit., note 334 above) erroneously believed that Edward's Leicestershire estate passed to the apothecary; the pedigree produced by him is defective and in parts clearly impossible. The estate, of nearly 1000 acres and eight messuages, was sold in 1750 to John Owsley of Hallaton, an apothecary.

[340] The Conyers of Walthamstow originated in Whitby and Scarborough. Tristram and Robert, two of Anthony Conyers of Bagdaile-hall's five sons, came south to find their fortunes. In this Tristram, at least, was eminently successful, for he built a capital messuage in Hoe Street, Walthamstow, and had estates in Lincolnshire and East Ham. Members of his family were William Conyers MD, who died of the plague in 1665, and Sir Gerard Conyers, governor of the Levant Company and director of the Bank of England.

[341] Holmes, op. cit., note 2 above, pp. 7, 11.

not all the professions are represented, at least four are to be found within the family of Thomas and Lewis Dickenson, apothecaries of Stafford.

The Dickensons' origins lay in a substantial Staffordshire yeoman family which, in 1575, was the tenant of a house in the manor of Acton Trussell, four miles south of Stafford. The century still had another seven years to run when the property was sold to the Dickensons.[342] Lewis's son, Lewis (a confusingly common name in the family), matriculated at St Alban's Hall, Oxford, in 1601, when he was seventeen, but this was the family's sole contact with the university world for well over a century. The Lewis of each succeeding generation inherited the small estate at Acton, until we come to the great-grandson. This particular Lewis and his wife Elizabeth died young, leaving their two boys, the inevitable Lewis and his younger brother Thomas, to be brought up by their grandfather.[343] As was proper, the elder son was guided in the ways of being a landowner, but Thomas was made an apothecary. Where he was trained is not known, but he was certainly practising in Stafford by 1707. Like his parents, Thomas did not live to middle age; both he and his wife were dead by 1721, and left two sons, another Lewis and another Thomas, to be brought up by their father's brother, Uncle Lewis, and his wife Mary.

It was decided that this youngest of the Lewis Dickensons was to be an apothecary like his father, and accordingly he travelled to Ashby-de-la-Zouch, Leicestershire, for a seven-year apprenticeship, starting on 1 September 1729 under John Mynors.[344] Before his time was finished, the young man, who must have been remarkably competent for his age, was recalled in August 1735, to deal with the problems that had arisen as a result of his Uncle Lewis's death the previous year. His Aunt Mary was now responsible for four young people, her own three, Lewis, Edward, and Mary, and her nephew Thomas. She received help from her brother, Thomas Ward, a banker in Fleet Street, London, but the person who increasingly and successfully organized the whole family was the young apothecary.

Whilst Lewis Dickenson had been living in Ashby, his younger brother Thomas had been packed off in the autumn of 1732 to Worcester to be trained as a grocer. Earlier, Thomas had been educated at Newport, Shropshire, by his father's cousin, John Dickenson, who, like his brother Joseph, subsequently entered the church.[345] John and

---

[342] *Victoria county history, Staffordshire*, Institute of Historical Research, 1959, vol. 5, pp. 12–14.

[343] The William Salt Library. Most of the information about the Dickenson family has been taken from the Hand-Morgan collection, which is not yet fully catalogued. On 10 February 1648, an indenture was made between William Goldsmith, yeoman, and Lewis Dickenson of Acton for the marriage of Goldsmith's daughter Jane and Lewis's son Lewis; Goldsmith supplying a £600 marriage portion and Dickenson lands and tenements. Litigation arose and there were law suits in 1649, 1687, 1689, 1690, and 1712, in which there was much useful recapitulation.

[344] PRO, Inland Revenue apprenticeship records, I.R./1/12, f. 1, premium £50. John Mynors was obviously a man who believed in frankness; he died on 26 June 1749, and had written on his mural monument in St Helen's church that he had ". . . by a successful practice carried on many years here enjoyed the pleasure of doing good, both to himself and those about him." He had a number of apprentices, as did Thomas Dickenson, including a boy from Ashby and another from London.

[345] John became vicar of Blymhill and was followed there by his son Samuel and his grandson John Horatio Dickenson. Samuel was a man of parts; he had a degree in law from St John's College, Cambridge, and a famous garden where he grew many aromatic Mediterranean plants collected when he travelled as tutor to Charles Darwin (1758–78), uncle to the famous zoologist. Joseph became rector of St Mary's, Stafford, and on 12 September 1772, he married William Withering to Helen Cooke, daughter of the town clerk. Joseph was followed at Stafford by his son Edward.

THE DICKENSONS OF ACTON TRUSSELL, STAFFORD, AND NEWPORT, SALOP

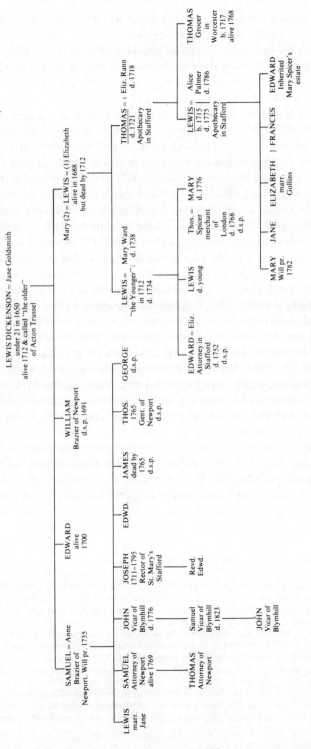

Compiled from MSS. at Wm. Salt library, Stafford, and Wills of members of the Dickenson family.

103

Joseph Dickenson were among the eight sons of Samuel; another, Samuel, became an attorney. By this time – early mid-eighteenth century – representatives of four professions were to be found in the family – and two trades.

Lewis took the guardianship of his young brother very seriously. Early in 1738, Thomas, living with Mr Edwards, grocer, in the High Street, Worcester, received a very terse and admonitory letter, ". . . you will receive about the same time two guineas sent by Martin the carrier. Your demand of twelve guineas put me upon looking whether so much was due to you, and upon enquiring found your letter of 21st. Feb. was in a very improper language. I will do everything I possibly can in my power to oblige and serve you but reckoning £5 per cent you are still outgone your allowance. I would have you take this into serious consideration for it is your own loss, and not lay out money as though you had twice the Income you have."

The year before, Lewis Dickenson had helped his Aunt Mary, who was rapidly failing, to place her eldest son Edward as an articled attorney's clerk with their father's cousin, the previously mentioned Samuel Dickenson of Newport. Edward's articles stated that Samuel was to ". . . instruct his clerk in the profession of law and practice of an attorney of the Court of Common Pleas at Westminster . . . as a Solicitor in the Courts of Equity and in conveyancy . . . and will take his clerk to London in term time to learn the method of managing and transacting the business of attorney and solicitor and at the end of the said five years at the request and cost of the said Edward Dickenson procure him to be admitted an attorney in the Court of Common Pleas."[346] It is not known if he ever practised in London, but, in any case, he was living at his house in Gaolgate, Stafford, at the time of his death in 1752. His brother-in-law, Thomas Spicer, citizen and haberdasher of London and husband of his sister Mary, had the thankless task of bringing order into Edward's affairs. There were problems with the Acton Trussell estate, which he had inherited, more trouble with another estate farther north in the county at Millmeece, and a very sizeable mortgage. At considerable cost to himself, Spicer sorted things out, the final act being the sale of Edward's house when Edward's widow married a Stafford surgeon and apothecary, Brooke Crutchley, in 1767.[347]

Spicer died the following year, and his will led to many furious letters and allegations between the Dickenson family and Spicer's brother John, a clergyman in Reading, in which Lewis was involved to the hilt.[348] The apothecary was no stranger to litigation; there was the case of Dickenson v. Clarke, which concerned a trespass at Cotonfield, and that of Dickenson v. Drakeford, in which he acted as the executor of

[346] Hand-Morgan collection, op. cit., note 343 above, MS. S.R. 249/6. Samuel was to find meat, drink, washing, and lodging, and to pay Edward £10 10s. at the end of his term, premium £105. The witnesses were Thomas Unett, ironmonger, and Lewis Dickenson, the apothecary. Young Edward did not join Samuel's law firm, possibly because Samuel's own son Thomas was the successor.

[347] Brooke, the son of John Crutchley of Hatherston, Warwickshire, had started his seven-year apprenticeship on Christmas Day 1732 with Edmund Seager, surgeon and apothecary, of the same town. Crutchley had at least three apprentices himself in Stafford between 1744 and 1760.

[348] Thomas Spicer had already let off his Reading house at £65 a year and also his bleaching ground there. John Spicer did some much-needed arithmetic and came up with the figures of £8,294 for his brother's assets and £8,460 for his commitments, which thus left no residue for John; equally disturbing was the fact that the London house John had been left in Fleet Street was in need of extensive repairs and adjoined a poor and noisy area. Mary Spicer departed from the fray and spent most of her last years in Bath, living for long periods with Lady Stanley.

Richard Drakeford of Forebridge, member of a well-known Staffordshire family.[349] Even more complicated was his involvement with the Palmers of Aston Hall outside Stafford. His wife's brother, John Palmer, had died intestate in 1766, leaving a widow and two infant daughters. As there was doubt as to Mrs Palmer's probity, the inheritance was put under the direction of the Court of Chancery, which appointed Lewis Dickenson receiver and manager of the rents and estates.

In the midst of such activity, he practised medicine and pharmacy and found time to be busy with civic affairs. He was mayor of Stafford from 1755 to 1759, and amongst his papers are lists of ale-house licences, constable's court papers, and accounts for the payments of electors. This busy life came to an end in July 1775, when he was just over sixty.

So lived the Dickensons. Not a family that was involved in national affairs, nor one that made a noteworthy mark in the academic world, but one which could certainly be described as professional and which was well known and respected in the west Midlands. The Dickensons are illustrative of those well-to-do families of yeoman status which proved a rich source for the consolidating professional corps. It is no less true of the minor gentry families that they proved a fine ground for recruitment.

Such a family was that of Septimus Bott (1646–1702), the son of Thomas Bott, an armigerous gentleman of modest pretensions at the family home of Dunstall-hall in the Forest of Needwood.[350] Thomas, dying in 1652, left his widow with six children, ranging in age from eleven to five, for whom provision had to be made. The estate of some 220 acres (and so probably only of the order of that of the Dickensons), was preserved intact for the eldest son John, who helped matters along by marrying into the landowning Wolferstan family. The other three boys had to fend for themselves, the youngest, Septimus, becoming an apothecary.

His apprentice-master is unknown, but Septimus took the step of obtaining the freedom of the London Society of Apothecaries by redemption in June 1670. He was still on the yeomanry list three years later, the probable year of his marriage to Joan, the widow of Thomas Pidgeon, alderman and apothecary of Coventry.[351] Septimus died in 1702, aged fifty-six, having outlived his brother John by sixteen years. It is apparent from his will that his thirty years' work in Coventry had done much to restore the family's fortunes. He owned not only his house in the Cross Cheaping but also lands in Warwickshire and Kent, and had arranged an advantageous marriage between his daughter Ann and Thomas, the son of the Reverend Michael Armestead of Waddington. No mention is made of the career of Septimus's elder son, but the apothecarial business was inherited by the second son, Thomas (1680–1739). It is assumed that Thomas, then twenty-two, had been trained by his father, though

[349] Matthew Drakeford, son of Richard, in 1731, was apprenticed to Thomas Addenbrooke (a Staffordshire man), citizen and apothecary of London. Twenty years later, Drakeford was practising in Cannock and taking apprentices himself.

[350] S. Shaw, *The history and antiquities of Staffordshire*, Wakefield, E. P. Publishing Co., 1976 (reprint), vol. 1, p. 111; R. Plot, *The natural history of Staffordshire*, Oxford, 1686. The Bott arms are engraved on the attached map; John Bott was a friend and correspondent of Robert Plot.

[351] In the church of Holy Trinity, Coventry, is a handsome marble monument to Thomas Pidgeon and his two wives, Elizabeth Foxley and Joan Foster née Greene. Pidgeon had four sons and a daughter, Elizabeth, who married John Dugdale, the eldest son of William of Blithe Hall; it was she who raised the monument.

THE BOTTS OF DUNSTALL AND COVENTRY

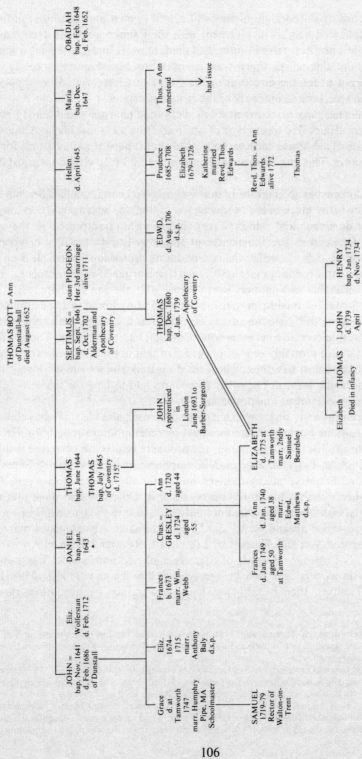

THOMAS BOTT = Ann
of Dunstall-hall
died August 1652

JOHN = 1641
bap. Nov. 1641
d. Feb. 1686
of Dunstall

Eliz.
Wolferstan
d. Feb. 1712

THOMAS
bap. June 1644

THOMAS
bap. July 1645
of Coventry
d. 1715?

DANIEL
bap. Jan.
1643
*

SEPTIMUS =
bap. Sept. 1646
d. Oct. 1702
Alderman and
Apothecary
of Coventry

Joan PIDGEON
Her 3rd marriage
alive 1711

Hellen
d. April 1645

Maria
bap. Dec.
1647

OBADIAH
bap. Feb. 1648
d. Feb. 1652

Grace
d. at
Tamworth
1747
marr. Humphry
Pipe, MA
Schoolmaster

Eliz.
1674–
1715
marr.
Anthony
Baly
d.s.p.

Frances
b. 1673
marr. Wm.
Webb

JOHN
Apprenticed
in
London
June 1693 to
Barber-Surgeon

THOMAS
bap. Dec. 1680
d. Jan. 1739
Apothecary
of Coventry

EDWD.
d. Aug. 1706
d.s.p.

Prudence
1685–1708

Thos. = Ann
Armestead

had issue

SAMUEL
1719–79
Rector of
Walton-on-
Trent

Chas. =
GRESLEY
d. 1724
aged
55

Ann
d. 1720
aged 44

ELIZABETH
d. 1775 at
Tamworth
marr. 2ndly
Samuel
Beardsley

Elizabeth
1679–1726
married
Revd. Thos.
Edwards

Revd. Thos. = Ann
Edwards

Katherine
married
Revd. Thos.
Edwards

Thomas

Frances
d. Jan. 1749
aged 50
at Tamworth

Ann
d. Jan. 1740
aged 38
marr.
Edwd.
Matthews
d.s.p.

Elizabeth
Died in infancy

THOMAS

JOHN
d. 1739
April

HENRY
bap. Jan. 1734
d. Nov. 1734

*It is thought Daniel was the father of John Butt, mercer of Burton-on-Trent. d. 1733.

106

possibly he had been to London for a short while.[352]

When he was nearing forty, Thomas married. His bride, Elizabeth Gresley, was related to him, as she was the granddaughter of Uncle John, who had inherited Dunstall-hall. John's daughter, Anne, had married Charles, the son of Sir Charles Gresley, baronet. The Gresleys of Drakelow were an important and powerful landed family in the counties of Stafford and Derby. Whilst it may have been thought unusual for a son of the Gresleys to have married a daughter of an impoverished minor gentleman, later generations would have decreed that the marriage between a Gresley daughter and a man who was indisputably involved in retail trade as an apothecary was totally inappropriate, not to say unacceptable. The shop counter does not seem to have caused social ostracism at that period.

Thomas was by no means ashamed of his own family, the Botts, as can be seen from his will made in 1734. He wished his eldest son John "... to be bred to the Law if qualified for such imployment". In the event, John was not put to the test, as he died within a few weeks of his father. The second son, Henry, predeceased his father, so that Thomas left no heir, a situation he had envisaged. He wrote in his will that, should his sons die under the age of twenty-one, then the residue of his real estate was to pass to his cousin John Bott of Burton-on-Trent, mercer, (son of his father's brother Daniel), and his male heirs, but if in default, it was bequeathed to his cousin Thomas Bott of Stratford-upon-Avon and his male heirs, "... it being my desire that the said estate should continue in the name of Bott."[353]

Elizabeth Bott (née Gresley, and soon to be Beardsley) would have been surprised and possibly indignant to have heard apothecaries described as "barely respectable" (p. 92), because apart from her husband there were at least five in her own family. Her father Charles, like his older brother Thomas (1668–1743), had been bound apprentice to wealthy City of London merchants; neither stayed on in the capital but returned to the country to live on their estates, Charles at Dunstan-hall with his wife Anne Bott, and Thomas at Nether Seale on the estate given to him by his mother.[354] Thomas's fifth son John (1711–83) married twice and had a large family. Two sons entered the church, another became an army officer, and two, James Henry (1751–?) and William Theophilus (1754–1826) Gresley became the apprentices of Walter Lyon and James Oldershaw, surgeons and apothecaries and men-midwives of Tamworth, who have already been mentioned (p. 31).[355] James Henry died young, but William

---

[352] PRO, PCC, Prob. 11 468 f. 20, February 1703. At the time of his death, he was an alderman of Coventry and his memorial in Holy Trinity proclaims him to have been a faithful supporter of the monarchy and the Church of England. Septimus's brother Thomas sent his son John to London in 1693 to be apprenticed to John Blankley, citizen and barber-surgeon. John did not take up his freedom but started a dynasty of apothecaries and surgeons in Stratford-upon-Avon.

[353] PRO, PCC, Prob. 11 697 f. 189, July 1739. John Bott, the mercer, was in fact dead at the time Thomas made his will in the autumn of 1734, having died the previous year, but he left five sons, Edward, John, Thomas, Daniel, and James.

[354] F. Madan, *The Gresleys of Drakelow*, William Salt Archaeological Society, 1898, vol. 19, pp. 95, 98–99.

[355] James Oldershaw had married Ruth Wilcockson, a relation of James Henry and William Theophilus Gresley's mother. Theophilus called in Oldershaw and Lyon to the confinement of his wife on 29 September 1781. When it was apparent that all was not well, William Withering was brought in on 5 October; matters did not improve and she was buried on the 26th. Allegations of neglect were brought against Withering. See Peck and Wilkinson, op. cit., note 306 above, p. 97.

Theophilus, like a distant cousin, Philip Gresley, became a member of the London Company of Surgeons.[356]

Families were clannish in the eighteenth century, and contact was maintained for generations between the spreading branches, so that it is no surprise to find marriages between first, second, and third cousins. The aunt of James and Theophilus, Elizabeth Gresley, married into the Gresleys of Bristol. She thereby became the second wife of a merchant, Henry, the sister-in-law of an Oxford MB, Robert (1696–1760) and of an apothecary, Francis (1708–91), and the daughter-in-law of another apothecary, Charles (1660–1735). Charles was the son of Thomas Gresley MA (Oxon.), royalist, tutor to the Earl of Clare's son, prebend of Worcester Cathedral, and a writer and translator of repute.[357] It is scarcely in dispute that the Gresleys were an upper-middle-class family, amongst whom were representatives of the landed gentry, clergy, attorneys, army surgeons, army officers, merchants, and apothecaries.

The detailed examination of the connexions of Septimus and Thomas Bott showed a not dissimilar pattern. Their antecedents were minor landowners; two of Thomas's sisters married clergymen, one set of cousins were mercers, another surgeons and apothecaries, a girl cousin married an MA who became a schoolmaster in Wolverhampton. It all provides an interesting commentary on provincial life in the first half of the eighteenth century. Landowner, merchant, parson, solicitor, and apothecary, their lives intermingled and they were on intimate terms with each other, a far cry from the nicely adjusted social stratigraphy of Victorian England. Lewis Dickenson and the two Botts were men of position and influence in their towns. Their opinions and help were sought by many sections of society. They had a close and familiar, not to say family, relationship with the local gentry, with London merchants and bankers, and with members of the well-recognized professions of the law and the church. One is forced to the conclusion that a man who participated in retail trade in the early and mid-eighteenth century was by no means condemned to social ostracism. Willan has made the suggestion that, ". . . it was the social snobbery of the Victorians that invented the tradesmen's entrance."[358]

Snobbery relating to retail trade does not seem to have had much weight with the two young men of non-conformist background, Richard Pulteney and James Taylor, when they were discussing the latter's future career. Taylor, when he was at the Northampton Academy in 1749, wrote, "I have been very uneasy with regard to my future employment in life and cannot think of any profession because of the close

[356] Both of them are to be found on the Surgeons' Lists for 1777, Philip as an army surgeon and Theophilus as living at Ashbourne. Two years later, the latter was in Tamworth, probably with Oldershaw, but after the death of his infant son in 1784, he moved away. After another short marriage, he became house-surgeon at the Liverpool Infirmary for twenty years; Philip Gresley (1751–1825), the son of an attorney, was more closely related to the Bristol Gresleys; he was an apprentice of Timothy Healy, surgeon and apothecary of Amersham for seven years, and was appointed to the 11th Dragoons in 1776.

[357] Madan, op. cit., note 354 above, p. 134. Charles Gresley, apothecary, became a burgess of Bristol in 1684 and built up a very successful practice. He married twice and fathered seven sons, three of whom entered the church, one became a physician, and two merchants. His next-to-youngest son Francis followed Charles in his apothecary's practice and was equally successful. Francis was the grandfather of Anthony Trollope's redoubtable mother, Fanny Milton, see J. Johnston, *The life, manners and travels of Fanny Trollope*, London, Constable, 1979, pp. 15, 25.

[358] T. S. Willan, *An eighteenth century shopkeeper, Abraham Dent of Kirkby Stephen*, Manchester University Press, 1970, p. 146.

PEDIGREE OF GRESLEY

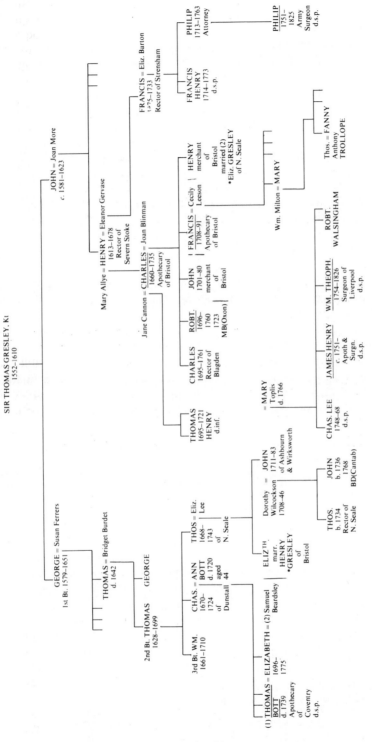

SIR THOMAS GRESLEY. Kt
1552-1610

GEORGE = Susan Ferrers
1st Bt. 1579-1651

JOHN = Joan More
c. 1581-1623

THOMAS = Bridget Burdet
d. 1642

GEORGE

Mary Allye = HENRY = Eleanor Gervase
1613-1678
Rector of Severn Stoke

FRANCIS = Eliz. Barton
1575-1733
Rector of Strensham

PHILIP
1713-1763
Attorney

2nd Bt. THOMAS
1628-1699

Jane Cannon = CHARLES = Joan Blinman
1660-1735
Apothecary of Bristol

FRANCIS
HENRY
1714-1773
d.s.p.

PHILIP
1751-1825
Army
Surgeon
d.s.p.

3rd Bt. WM.
1661-1710

CHAS. = ANN
1670-   BOTT
1724   d. 1720
of   aged
Dunstall 44

THOS. = Eliz.
1668-   Lee
1743
of
N. Seale

THOMAS
1695-1721
HENRY
d.inf.

CHARLES
1695-1761
Rector of
Blagden

ROBT.
1696-
1760
MB(Oxon)

JOHN
1701-80
merchant
of
Bristol

FRANCIS = Cecily
1708-91   Leeson
Apothecary
of Bristol

HENRY
merchant
of
Bristol
married (2)
*Eliz. GRESLEY
of N. Seale

ELIZTH
marr.
HENRY
*GRESLEY
of
Bristol

Dorothy = JOHN
Wilcockson 1711-83
1708-46   of Ashbourn
          & Wirksworth

= MARY
Toplis
d. 1766

Wm. Milton = MARY

Thos. = FANNY
Anthony
TROLLOPE

(1) THOMAS = ELIZABETH = (2) Samuel
BOTT   1696-   Beardsley
d. 1739   1775
Apothecary
of
Coventry
d.s.p.

THOS,
b. 1734
Rector of
N. Seale

JOHN
b. 1736
1768
BD(Cantab)

CHAS. LEE
1748-68
d.s.p.

JAMES HENRY
c. 1751-
Apoth &
Surgn.
d.s.p.

WM. THEOPH.
1754-1826
Surgeon of
Liverpool
d.s.p.

ROBT.
WALSINGHAM

application necessary in the pursuit; and as to a trade I am sure I could not support the confinement of a shop, nor bear to sit behind a counter from one weeks end to another." Seven weeks later, he enlarged on the subject, "If you ask what employment I should chose myself . . . of all the different mechanic business . . . or employment which go under the denomination of trades I think I should prefer that of a 'Retail Draper', it seems such a neat cleanly business and what prejudices me in its favour is the good hours they keep, the leisure for reading and improving the mind, and the liberty which it affords to sanctify the Sabbath." In the end, he decided to become a grazier, ". . . it is genteel employment and affords much spare time . . . I dont on any account intend to mingle farming with it which I am prodigiously aversed to."[359]

Social snobbery was not invented by the Victorians, but they inherited and embellished it. If one were to place a date for the origin of the denigration of retail trade, one might hazard that of 1750. The three London medical organizations enacted three far-reaching statutes in the middle years of the eighteenth century: (1) the Surgeons' Company's by-laws of 1748, which forbade the election to the Court of ". . . anyone who practised as an apothecary or followed any other trade or occupation besides the profession or business of a surgeon.";[360] (2) the College of Physicians' statute of 1758, which stated that no one who had ever practised as an apothecary or kept open shop was eligible under any circumstances for election to the fellowship;[361a] (3) the Society of Apothecaries, by 1774, felt it was time for its higher echelons to dissociate in some degree from retail trade and so resolved that only those apothecaries practising medicine would be allowed on the livery.[361b]

An interesting comparison may be made with the rapidly increasing interest in plantsmanship and the rise of the nurseryman in the late seventeenth and eighteenth centuries. On 12 August 1740, a sermon was preached by Charles Lamotte DD, chaplain to the Prince of Wales, "at a meeting of Gentlemen Florists, and Gardeners" at Stamford. Harvey has written,

The coming together of gentlemen florists and gardeners was a symptom of great significance. . . . The archives of the Ancient Society of York Florists, complete from its foundation in 1768, show by the actual signatures on the roll the almost complete coverage of society by the keen interest in flowers . . . the membership included knights, baronets and lords of great estates as well as professional men and minor shopkeepers. . . . It is known that the Exeter society, after a good start, became divided by the new snobbery early in the 19th. century, and an attempt was made – though happily defeated – to remove the tradesmen from its ranks.[362]

The successful legislation of the London medical bodies against retail trade nurtured this snobbery until such ridiculous statements as the following could be made in 1811: "Mr Cunnington's account of the different articles displayed very considerable powers of mind, as well as originality, and was conveyed in a language and manner peculiarly his own; and left us in admiration of acquirements so rarely met with in men of his rank and calling, who affected no other character than that of a respectable tradesman. . . ."[363] Or, in the mid-nineteenth century: "He lived to show

[359] Linnean Library, Pulteney letters, 3 March [1749], 22 April 1749, 14 July 1749.
[360] Wall, op. cit., note 24 above, p. 54.
[361] Wall, Cameron, and Underwood, op. cit., note 8 above, vol. 1, (a) p. 189, (b) p. 188.
[362] John Harvey, *Early nurserymen*, Chichester, Phillimore, 1974, p. 37.
[363] R. H. Cunnington, *From antiquary to archaeologist*, Princes Risborough, Shire Publications, 1975, p. 92. William Cunnington was a fine archaeologist of the latter part of the eighteenth century, who was ins-

how much of the coarser duties of this busy World may be undertaken by a man of quick sensibility without impairing the finer sense of the beautiful in nature and in art. . . ."[364]

The denigration of the apothecary and the delicate drawing away of skirts from anything that smacked of retail trade was in full swing by 1800. Richard Smith junior, surgeon of the Bristol Infirmary from 1796 to 1843, wrote a valuable account of medical practice in Bristol. Of the apothecary at the turn of the eighteenth century, he wrote,

> About the year 1793 there were in Bristol 35 professed Apothecaries and 20 Surgeons, amongst the latter there were 8 or 10 who considered it to be infra. dig. to put 'Apothecary' upon their doors, yet the greatest part among these practised Physic and dispensed medicines. Amongst the Infirmary list Mr Godfrey Lowe and Mr Noble confined themselves to Surgery. But Mr Yeatman acted as an Apothecary and dispensed his medicines. . . . Mr Allard although he held himself very high and was very indignant at the idea of being otherwise than 'A Surgeon' – yet he not only practised Physic but was actually known by the name of 'Shop'. He however had his Bills for medicines made out in the name of his Apprentice and pretended that it was a perquisite of his 'young man' – but the fact was that every shilling . . . went into his own pocket.[365]

These curious ideas of the last two hundred years have been extrapolated backwards, and the belief has been, and still is by the majority, held that there was an almost absolute rupture between the professional physician and the trading apothecary throughout their mutual histories. Wherever a community or a family is studied in detail, this has not proved to be the case. Of the Bromfields of London it has been written,

> It was then [the Victorian era] strongly held that in some mysterious way trade was denigrating . . . never could it be intermingled with the true professions of the church, medicine and the law. In this country it has never been denied that a family might start from humble origins but in the upward climb all such associations had to be ruthlessly discarded. Yet here is a family which remained in close and intimate terms with each other, who covered a wide spectrum of social position, from an apothecarial shopkeeper, a druggist and tea-man to a barrister of Gray's Inn, an MD of Oxford, and a surgeon to the royal household.[366]

This conclusion was borne out by Dr Zuck's researches into John Mervyn Nooth. He discovered that John's father, Henry, apothecary of Sturminster Newton, Dorset, was the son of the Reverend Nooth, prebendary of Wells. Henry married Biddy, the daughter of John Mervin, apothecary, and probably Nooth's apprentice-master. Mervin had sent his son, Edward, to Balliol in 1728, where he obtained a BA. In his turn, Henry sent his son, John Mervin, to Edinburgh and then on the "grand tour"; he purchased a commission for his other son, Henry, in a fashionable regiment. The younger Henry married into the landed gentry, his wife being the female survivor of the extinct baronetcy of Vavasour of Spaldington. This background would have been

---

trumental in liberating the new subject from the thraldom of the classics. He was a draper who later became a successful wool merchant.

[364] *Chronicles of Cannon Street*, published privately by Messrs. Joseph Travers & Sons, [n.d. ?1957], p. 20. This is a reference to William Smith, citizen and grocer of the Sugar Loaf, Cannon Street, London, reformer and first avowed non-conformist to take the oath in the House of Commons.

[365] F. H. Rawlings, 'The decline of the apothecary in Bristol', a paper read at the British Society for the History of Pharmacy conference at Bristol in 1979; it was extracted from the second volume of Richard Smith's 'Memoirs of the Infirmary'.

[366] Burnby and Whittet, op. cit., note 178 above, p. 9.

assigned to a physician without question.[367]

With this evidence before us, it is not surprising to find such county families as the Turvilles, the Herricks, and the Dixies of Leicestershire, the Parkyns and the Scroops of Nottinghamshire, the Meynells and the Bagshaws of Derbyshire figuring in the apprenticeship records both in London and the provinces.

[367] D. Zuck, 'The provincial apothecary', *Pharm. Hist.*, 1978, **8**: no. 2, unpaginated. Dr Zuck wrote, "During my researches on Nooth I began to have doubts about the validity of the picture of the provincial apothecary painted by such writers as Lester King. . . .".

CONCLUSION

Dempster, in a challenging article on John Hunter, has shown that "Attitudes to Mr Hunter, like propaganda, become repetitive so that the calumnies, once started, continue and few in the surgical world have doubted or cared whether they had substance or not." Again and again, men have written that he was "failing in scholarship", "did not bother to read books very much", was "hampered by a defective education", or had "a want of logical accuracy in his reasonings", all of which can be traced back to his first (1794) detractor, Jesse Foot. Dempster showed these parrot-like judgements to be manifestly untrue, and that Hunter was indeed a "thinking man", that "If John is to be denied the title of scholar because of his contempt for Latin and Greek and the Oxbridge set-up of the eighteenth century, we must place Darwin also in the ranks of the non-scholar."[368] Thus have a famous man's scholarship and powers of original thought been almost irremediably traduced, and in like manner has a whole professional group been denigrated over the years. Only a careful study of the lives of these people, the apothecaries of the seventeenth and eighteenth centuries, can redress the balance.

Trease has demonstrated that the lack of attention to English records has led to erroneous ideas about English pharmacy.[369] Living in an age that is conditioned to exact definitions and the legal protection of titles, it is difficult for us to project ourselves into a period when people were careless of such niceties. We have placed our own present-day interpretations on a title, and, as a result, have for long obscured pharmaceutical and medical history. Several workers have suspected that there was little difference, if any, between the so-called apothecary and the so-called surgeon of the period under review and even later, but proof was only forthcoming with the abstraction and subsequent analysis of all the medical personnel from the Inland Revenue apprenticeship records of the eighteenth century. During the century from 1660 to 1760, all branches of medicine widened their experience and expertise. It was even apparent to a contemporary, R. Campbell, who in 1747 said: "There is such a Connexion between the several Branches of Physic, that it is almost impossible for a Person to be Master of any one of them without a superficial Knowledge of all the rest. The Physician should know something of the Surgeon's Business, and he of the Doctor's, and the Apothecary of both."[370]

Financial considerations, in any case, forced many medical practitioners into a non-specialist practice. There is, nevertheless, an important exception to this general statement – the surgeons appointed to the voluntary hospitals. The hospital could supply them with so much surgical work that they could practise as that rarity, the "pure" surgeon. In London, the medieval hospitals of St Bartholomew and St Thomas were joined by the mid-eighteenth century by the Westminster (1719), Guy's (1725), St

---

[368] W. J. Dempster, 'Hunter the Scholar', *Wld Med.*, 1975, 87–96.

[369] Trease, op. cit., note 1 above, pp. 11–16.

[370] R. Campbell, *The London tradesman*, London, T. Gardiner, 1747; reprinted, Newton Abbot, David & Charles, 1969, p. 52.

George's (1733), the London (1740), and the Middlesex (1745) hospitals. Soon, a numerically small but powerful and very wealthy corpus of hospital surgeons grew up in the capital. In the provinces, the voluntary hospital was a slightly later and noticeably smaller development, and so the highly esteemed hospital surgeon was of a correspondingly later and less luxuriant growth. There were, however, twelve such hospitals in existence by 1755, which, it is estimated, housed around a thousand beds. In addition to its surgeons and physicians, each hospital had a resident apothecary, but the total numbers were so small it is not thought that they had an effect on the evolution of the profession.

The apothecary, in common with all vital institutions, varied in his function and practice through the centuries, changing his role with the demands of society and science. It is inaccurate to regard him as a dispensing doctor, or as a pharmacist with a busy counter-practice, making the occasional domiciliary visit or call on his physician's coffee house. In the years centring on 1700, he was physician and surgeon and pharmacist and retail grocer. As the years went by, he turned more and more to the practice of medicine. This is not surprising. Gregory King, in 1688, estimated that the population of England and Wales was five and a half millions, and the survey of London as a result of the Act of 1694 has given a figure of nearly 124,000 for the ninety-seven parishes within the walls and the thirteen outside; quite obviously the 114 members of the College of Physicians could not cope with numbers of that order.[371] As Trail has pointed out, the two English universities had inexplicably and regrettably failed in their duty. They were "... slow in adapting themselves to Continental methods of medical training which were attracting young men of good families.... Students were few; only 172 graduated in the 17th century, a lamentably small number in view of the growing population."[372] He was equally critical of the College of Physicians, "... it took the College authorities a long time to follow Harvey's advice and to admit that every physician must be at all times something of an empiric.... They should [have], much earlier than they did, ... copied the worthy example of the experimenting apothecaries, who took a much more practical view of the advances possible under the stimulus of the Royal Society."

The need and chances were there and the apothecary-surgeon took them, in which he was actively encouraged by his local authorities, who needed to implement the Poor Law Acts by those means available to them. The experience gained by this typically English medical practitioner was considerable long before the advent of the voluntary hospitals. His was a practical training for a practical subject, which, despite all jibes, paid off handsomely and laid the basis for the work of such fine physicians as William Withering, or surgeon-apothecaries-turned-physicians such as Edward Jenner.

The long-held views on the positions of the apothecary and surgeon in society without doubt require very considerable adjustment. Unequivocally, a man who possessed a medical degree was held to be a gentleman, who had nothing to do with the lowly apprenticeship system, and yet the records show otherwise. William Chambers of Hull, MD of Leiden (1724), Gilbert Heathcote of Derbyshire and London, MD of Padua (1688), and George Vaux of Reigate, MD of Leiden (1704) all took

[371] L. S. King, *The medical world of the eighteenth century*, Chicago University Press, 1958, p. 18; *London inhabitants within the walls*, op. cit., note 160 above, p. xx.

[372] R. R. Trail, 'Physicians and apothecaries in the seventeenth century', *Pharm. J.*, 1962, **188**: 206, 207.

their apprentices.[373] The last two men were Quakers, which debarred them from the English universities and accounts for the fact that George Vaux's brother Isaac, son George, nephew Isaac, and grandson George all became members of either the old Barber-Surgeons' Company or the new Surgeons' Company. It is doubtful if their social standing was any less than their father's or brother's.

The popular estimate of the provincial apothecary also needs a reassessment. He would seem not to have been the ignoramus so often believed. Willan has noted that Abraham Dent had much wider interests than those confined to a little market town such as Kirkby Stephen, and suggested that, "... if more were known about the Abraham Dents, eighteenth century England might appear less bucolic and less provincial."[374] Study of the Botts and the Dickensons certainly bears out this tentative conclusion. They were no strangers to London, and their contacts, both personal and for business, mostly through the widely spreading network of the immediate family and cousins to the second and third degree, are to be found in the towns and cities of the Midlands and that Mecca of fashion, Bath. They travelled more widely than is often thought. Mary Spicer and her husband moved between Stafford, Reading, and London; she was visited in Bath by her cousin Lewis and his wife and the old Rector, Joseph Dickenson (who caused problems by leaving his nightshirt behind), whilst Thomas Pidgeon and Septimus Bott both had professional ties with the London Society of Apothecaries.

The apothecary played an important civic role. Thomas Pidgeon was mayor of Coventry, and his son-in-law an alderman; Lewis Dickenson was mayor of Stafford and was involved in many of the town's activities; neither was this unusual. Several of the apothecaries of Chester became mayors of that city, the Joshua Bryans, junior and senior, were mayors of South Molton no less than five times between 1753 and 1810, and the famous William Franceys was mayor of Derby in 1697, 1699, and 1700, to be followed by his son Henry. Thomas Ryves, "pharmacopola" was town clerk of Hastings at the time of his death in 1691, in which position he was followed by Peter Fiott, "doctor in phisick".[375] Derry of Bath carried out research into the mayors of that town, and has come to the conclusion "... that families influential in corporation affairs either originated with apothecaries or sooner or later produced apothecaries among their members."[376]

At the same time, apothecaries were keenly interested in the developing sciences, in particular those that impinged on their own profession. They were in the forefront of the popular interest in natural history; the physic garden at Chelsea was of international fame, and it is probably true to say that no man had a wider connexion in the botanical world than James Petiver FRS. John Haughton FRS was sufficiently well thought of by the Royal Society to be invited to sit on the committee that had been set up to investigate the state of agriculture in England.

[373] William Chambers, who described himself as "Surgeon, etc" in the indentures, took as apprentice Ralph Darling, who subsequently became his son-in-law. In 1710, Joshua Fiddel of Leeds went as an apprentice to Gilbert Heathcote in Chesterfield. Richard Smith was apprenticed to George Vaux for seven years from 29 September 1711.

[374] Willan, op. cit., note 358 above, p. 146.

[375] 'Hastings and district', *Pharm. J.*, 1964, **194**: 651.

[376] W. Derry, 'Notes on the apothecaries of Bath', typescript deposited with the British Society for the History of Pharmacy, p. 1. Copy in author's possession.

It has been suggested that the apothecary's shop was in fact a health-centre in miniature. Roberts has said, "The apothecary shop was a focal point of the medical scene of the day [early seventeenth century]. It was tending to become a medical centre with, often, a team consisting of a physician, a surgeon, an empiric and an old woman who acted as a midwife. They relied on the apothecary, his shop, and his dispensing skills to keep the team going."[377] *If* this were the case – and it is not impossible – the reasons for the support that the apothecary received from the general populace are obvious, and equally obvious are some of the causes underlying the physician's jealousy. This focal point was no shop in the sense of a modern help-yourself store or seedy corner shop where dubious transactions took place at the back door. In any case, such research as has been carried out on retail trade in the eighteenth century indicates that the disparagement of the shopkeeper may well be a Victorian accretion to an idea which had begun to emerge some seventy years earlier, a view which has of recent years been enhanced by a modern belief that medical ethics and commerce, that is to say the "profit motive", are incompatible: the trader is a putative rogue, thus the apothecary must have been made of lesser clay than his medical colleagues.[378] The time has been more than ripe for a reappraisal of the apothecary, his life-style, his background and status, and his function as tailored by the social demands of his period.

[377] R. S. Roberts, 'Current problems: seventeenth century parallel', *Pharm. J.*, 1969, **202**: 38.

[378] The Parrys and Holloway see the Apothecaries' Act of 1815 as retrogressive because it placed the control of general practice under the jurisdiction of the Society of Apothecaries, a mercantile company, and thus degraded the general practitioner. N. and J. Parry, *The rise of the medical profession: a study in collective social mobility*, London, Croom Helm, 1976; S. W. F. Holloway, 'The Apothecaries' Act: a reinterpretation', *Med. Hist.*, 1966, **10**: 107–29, 221–236; J. K. Crellin, 'Sociology and the professions', *Pharm. J.*, 1977, **218**: 199.

INDEX

128